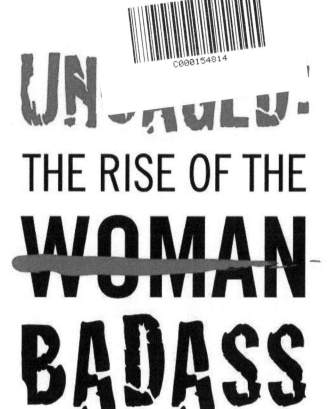

UN~~CAGED~~:

THE RISE OF THE

~~WOMAN~~

BADASS

Compiled and Published by
Michelle Catanach

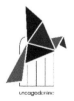

uncagedonline

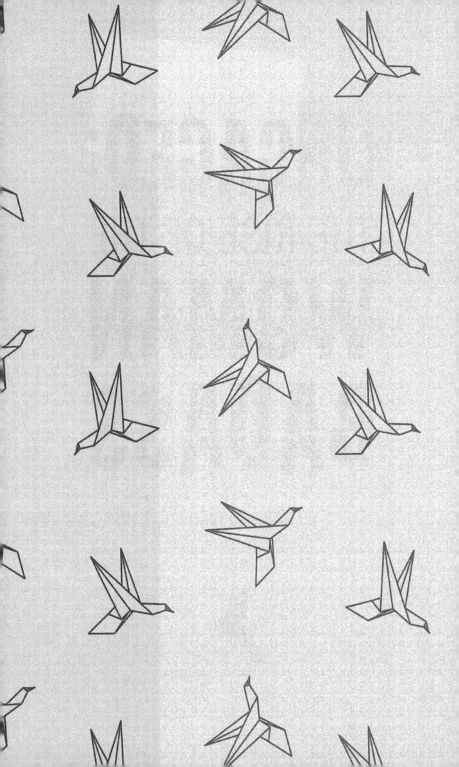

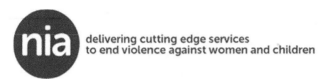

nia delivering cutting edge services
to end violence against women and children

Nia is a charity working on all forms of violence against women and girls. It has been operative since 1975 and mainly works in North and East London, it supports around 2,000 women and girls a year. Nia's services include:

- East London Rape Crisis
- Independent sexual violence advocates
- Independent domestic violence advocates
- IRIS – a programme working with GPs to improve awareness and referrals about domestic violence
- Play Therapy for children who have witnessed violence between parents or carers
- The London Exiting Advocacy project for women exiting prostitution
- Specialist refuges – one for women affected by sexual exploitation and one for women with problematic substance use (often as a coping strategy for violence and abuse they have suffered)
- Huggett women's centre

In addition, nia will also stand up for women and women's services and provide data, information, research, reports and evidence about women's experiences of male violence and trying to access support.

www.niandingviolence.org.uk

twitter @niaending_VAWG

Nia registered charity number 1037072

All royalties from the sale of this book will be donated to nia

Praise for *Uncaged: The Rise of the Badass*

'This is raw, honest, powerful, and often painful to read. But it is so necessary to hear these voices, those heart-breaking and at the same time heart-warming stories, that we usually don't hear anywhere often enough. I loved it and emerged from reading utterly awestruck, and with so much love, pride and admiration for the endurance and strength of these women - which shines through in every word of their stories' *Daniela Abinashi, Criminology Researcher*

'These stories bravely go deep into wounding and share with us the powerful path of transformation we all have available and which is empowered by this kind of conscious and supportive sharing among the female collective. The sharing of these women's challenging stories provides a healing mirror for our own and a guide for positive growth empowered by women who have gone before. A very important book for anyone on a healing journey' *Alice Bird, Actress*

'This powerful and timely book and the stories told by 26 badass women provide the perfect fuel to ignite the fire and fan the flames to help women free themselves from 'too muchness' and/or 'not enoughness.' These courageous women speak their authentic truth to provide the opening for us to heal. Read this book now (as life is too dang short!) and soak in the raw inspiration to be YOU, uniquely you. We can and must rebel from thousands of years of oppression and live fully now, to pave the way for future generations.' *Tanya Mark, Body Image Movement Global Ambassador www.tanyamark.com*

'*Uncaged: The Rise of the Badass* is a must read for anyone looking to be moved and inspired by authentic stories of the triumph of the female spirit. As twenty-six women share their unique stories of finding their strength and moving from living in darkness to shining in their own light, the reader is taken for a beautiful ride where the message is clear and powerful. Women have faced unbelievable barriers to freedom. Yet the indomitable nature of our hearts and will, as detailed through the authors' stories, leads to the unmistakable truth that we are powerful, we are strong, we can rise from trauma to healing and from adversity to strength and success' *Sindy Warren, author, yogi, lawyer www.yogaforyourbestlife.com*

'This book is a must read, I was totally drawn in from the start, I couldn't put it down and I could relate with many of the chapters either from my own experiences or from now connecting with people who have opened up to me about their lives and stories. I think this book will inspire and help many women and to let them know that they aren't alone, this is truly a book to read. Well done Michelle for putting it together, your story and the others were so heartfelt, thank you for opening yourselves up to the world to help others, what an amazing thing to do. Extraordinary women, thank you' *Amanda Skinner*

To our rising girls, navigating the complexities of the human world: you are *more* than enough.

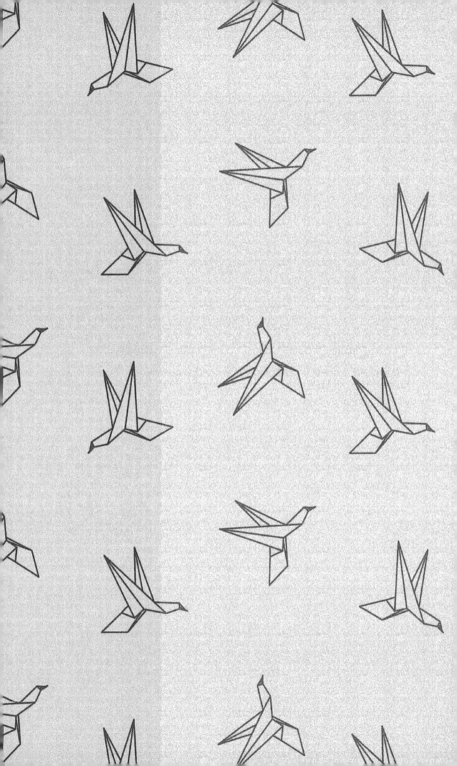

Contents

Introduction

For too long women have been treated less than.
Violated.
Abused.
Shamed.
Silenced.
Denied our basic human rights.

We've carried wounds, and stories from the past.
Burdened by labels, our pain hidden beneath a mask.
We've waged war within ourselves, and each other.
Told that we're too much, yet not enough.

We learned to please, to give away our power.
To bury our truth.
To hide our gifts and dim our light.
To tame the wild woman inside.

Until now.

The world is craving more.
More truth.
More vulnerability.
More authenticity.
More love.
More pleasure.

More connection.
More intimacy.

More women willing to show up as their perfectly imperfect messy selves.

More women willing to uncage themselves from the stories of the past and live with passion, purpose, integrity and freedom.

More women reclaiming their power and owning their darkness as well as the light.

More women rising together to create positive change in the world through truth, authenticity and an indestructible knowing that women are worthy and deserving of so much more.

When we rise our children rise. And *that* is how we change the world.

This book is part-memoir, part self-help, taking you on your own journey of insight, exploration and self-discovery so that you too can awaken to your truth and uncage the wild woman inside.

Freedom

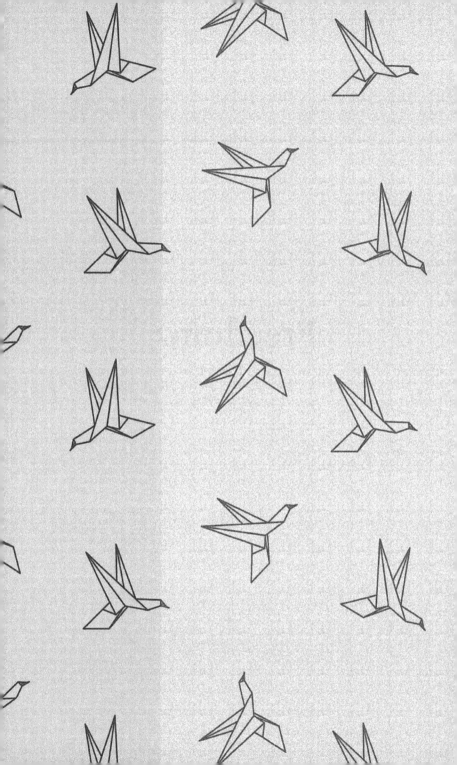

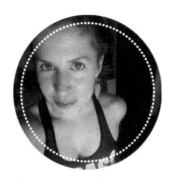

Swallowing My Demons
By Michelle Catanach

'Emancipate yourself from mental slavery. None but ourselves can free our minds' ~ Bob Marley

Have you ever wanted to die?

I'm not talking about wishing the ground would open up and swallow you in one of those excruciatingly embarrassing moments.

I mean *real* death. The kind when you honestly, genuinely don't want to live anymore. The kind when you deliberately with all intents and purposes attempt suicide. Not as a cry for help or to seek attention but because you have an almost palpable belief that the world would be a happier and better place without your worthless existence.

I did back when I was a mere 19 years old.

I remember that night as if it were yesterday, out drinking with friends in our regular haunt. It was that period in my life when I spent every night out boozing for fear of missing out, alcohol filling the void of what was an otherwise unexciting life. I didn't even have hobbies. I would wake up, go to work then to the pub. And I would continue this pattern every single day. Wash, rinse, repeat.

That night I was drunk. Booze made me a more fun and exciting person to be around, helping me lose my inhibitions and create a mask of confidence. And it helped me to take my mind off the emptiness I felt inside.

I was grieving that night, or at least that's how it felt. The loss of my ex after yet another volatile breakup had left me in a state of mourning.

I remember drinking copious amounts of vodka to hide my sadness. I was free of him so should have been celebrating, not drowning my sorrows. He was a complete bastard. Everyone told me so. Yet I didn't see it. I didn't want to. More than two years of torment and manipulation meant I was codependent and needy, convinced that I was nothing without him. Believed that I needed him to survive.

I was laughing on the outside, flirting with anyone with a pulse, yet crying on the inside, the voices and insecurities getting stronger the more inebriated I became.

The walk home was long and lonely without him by my side, yet the torment and abuse would have been unbearable if he was. I trudged through puddles, the rain drowning me and leaving me looking scruffy and bedraggled. I looked old for my 19 years. The way I walked, the clothes I wore and the pained expression set on my face, far removed from the vibrant and happy girl I'd once been.

I found myself calling him, begging him to take me back, sobbing as he screamed a torrent of abuse and profanities down the phone.

He was right.

I *was* a slag. A nutcase. A whore.

No one wanted me. Why would they? Even my family were ashamed and embarrassed by me.

At least *he* had wanted me. He had pitied me and taken the burden off someone else by being with me. He'd done the world a favour, taken one for the team. But even he had walked away. He couldn't bear the burden any longer.

At least that is what he had me believe.

I felt so alone. I didn't have anyone to talk to. I'd spent so many years thinking that showing emotion and asking for help was a weakness that I didn't know how to talk about my feelings, instead clamming up and pretending that everything was ok while bottling it all up inside. Until I could hold it in no longer, that is, and someone would find themselves on the receiving end of my rage.

And the truth was I missed him. I *needed* him. Without him I was nothing. He gave me a reason to wake up every morning even if it meant crying myself to sleep by bedtime.

A Dark Decision

I remember reaching home, swaying as I a fumbled around for my door key, tear-stained and bleary eyed. I staggered down the hallway and into the kitchen, the gaudy green and orange cupboards illuminated in the moonlight.

At this point, I wasn't thinking anything. I knew what I had to do. It had been an easy decision to make. I didn't even consider the outcome. What would it matter; I'd be dead.

The house was eerily silent as I opened the kitchen cupboard where I knew a stash of pills were stored. My hand blindly grappled around in the dark, rattling condiments and tins as I reached to the back of the cupboard. I pulled out whatever I could find.

And I took them. One by one. Rapidly pushing my feelings of self-loathing, loss and loneliness down with every swallow. Praying, *praying* that whatever they were, they would work.

I don't know how many I took. I don't even know what I was taking. I didn't care. I simply focused on the task at hand.

And then I went to bed.

The Aftermath

I awoke dazed and confused, my head throbbing as the room spun. I vomited into a pint glass that was on the floor beside my bed, initially impressed with myself that I'd avoided spewing on the carpet.

Then it hit me, like a juggernaut at 100mph.

I was still alive.

To this day I will never forget the wave of disappointment engulf my entire body as I realised that my attempt to end it all had failed. All the feelings of hurt, pain, hatred and despair came flooding in like a tsunami, leaving me in a crumpled, sobbing heap on my bed. I felt like I was grieving all over again. Angry at the world. Angry at myself.

Of course I carried on like nothing had happened, leaving the house that morning, my mum ranting as I left, affirming everything I already knew about me being a useless waste of space. Me being late for work with what she believed was simply yet another hangover only added more fuel to her ever-burning flame.

I called in sick at work then spent two hours sitting on the swing in a child's playground, head in hands, routinely vomiting as my body desperately tried to expel the toxins.

No one knew what I'd done. In fact it took several years before I confessed to anybody.

I'd like to say that this experience woke me up, that I saw that I had a second chance in life. Something to live for. That I would radically transform and live out my soul's desires.

But it didn't. It was simply another chapter in a profoundly troubled life that seemed to spiral downwards as soon as I turned 16.

In fact, I got back with my ex after that night. We even moved in together, the start of six months of emotional bullying, the odd black-eye and bruised ribs. I went to work struggling to make ends meet while he bummed around watching porn and smoking pot all day.

Such was his power, his control, that everyone thought it was me. *I* was the problem. They saw a crazed, nagging girlfriend. What they didn't see was the powerless girl reacting to whispered threats and muttered taunts while he acted like the innocent, downtrodden boyfriend to the outside world.

I despised the guy but felt too weak to leave. I fell into a deeper depression, stuck in a limbo of not wanting to be at home and not wanting to be at work. Not wanting to be anywhere. Until one day I found myself with my hands around his throat, squeezing it tight, desperately trying to rid myself of this nightmare that I'd found myself living in.

For a moment I wanted to kill him. To end the torture.

I only stopped because a voice in my head told me so; he wasn't worth a prison sentence.

It was then that I knew I had to leave.

This triggered several years of self-destructive behaviour as I found solace in anything that would make me feel validated, loved or simply numb the pain.

Drugs, excessive drinking, countless one-night-stands, toxic friendships, extreme dieting, binge eating, laxative addiction, rebounding from one job to another, clinging on to lousy men while pushing away any chance of happiness. Anything that gave me a hit of dopamine while supporting a deeply embedded unconscious belief that I wasn't worthy enough.

I was a far cry from the straight A student from my school days who'd had so much promise and potential. And a far greater cry from the baby given the spiritual name of Joy for the delight she would supposedly bring to other people's lives.

The Return of Joy

I didn't know who I was or even who I was supposed to be. For a long time, I was lost.
So I made the best decision of my life: I went travelling.

Travelling had been a dream of mine for years, but I'd been so sucked in by my boozy lifestyle and toxic relationships that I didn't have the motivation –or self-belief -to go ahead and do it, only lame excuses not to.

Then I met Steve who'd already travelled the world twice. He took me on holiday to Cambodia, and after being so touched by the experience, it was then that I knew: I *had* to travel.

I asked Steve to join me. Reluctantly he agreed. Our first year together had been hell (for him). So convinced was I that he was just like all the others that I constantly tried to provoke him to prove my belief that all men were arseholes. In reality I was the aggressor, often violently lashing out after too much drink. He, of course, never retaliated.

Travelling was the making of me, and while it forces many couples apart, it brought Steve and me closer together. Away from the people, places and situations that triggered my insecurities, I was able to see things clearly.

I finally understood love, compassion and humanity. I learned how the world actually worked, witnessing genuine innate happiness in people with materially poor lives. I observed pure joy and gratitude despite apparent hardship and often traumatic pasts.

I realised that Steve wasn't like all the others and that he was, in fact, a decent bloke (and double brownie points for putting up with so much of my shit when most men would simply walk away). But most of all, I made peace with myself. I accepted myself and no longer felt ashamed of who I was.

When I stood on top of a relatively small mountain in Australia's Warrumbungle National Park on my 26th birthday, for the first time in 10 years, I felt free. I had finally left the bullshit of the past behind.

Joy had come home.

Spiralling Back Into The Shadow

Following that day life became pretty phenomenal. I overcame eating issues and effortlessly shed a load of weight. I drastically cut down on the booze. I discovered hobbies and a passion for learning. I cycled from London to Paris and ran my first half marathon, feats that before I wouldn't have considered trying. I had more travelling adventures. I attracted some amazing people into my life, forming deep and meaningful connections and my career, which had always been a non-starter, soared. And remember Steve? Against all the odds we got married (in Vegas!) and now have two gorgeous children (and this despite my resistance and belief that I didn't deserve kids).

Then I followed my dream. I left work to have baby number 2, set up a business then BOOM! All of the crap about me not being good enough, stuff that I thought I'd overcome but had in fact locked away in the shadowy depths of my mind, reared its ugly head.

I felt my life spiralling downwards again. All those old feelings of shame and self-loathing were creeping back. I felt like a failure. I was a terrible mother. A neglectful wife. And my business was a sinking ship weighed down by mounting debt.

I started drinking more alcohol than normal, bingeing on junk and not taking care of myself.
I retreated into myself, pushing people away and felt ashamed for imagining life without my kids. The stress and overwhelm was all consuming, and I didn't recognise the person I was anymore. I only knew I didn't like who I was becoming.

My Awakening

Then it happened. My 3-year-old daughter hit me. The red mist set in. And at that moment all my pent up frustration came out as I picked her up by her shoulders and shouted aggressively in her face, took her to her room and threw her - like a rag doll - onto her bed.

When I saw her sobbing inconsolably, pleading with me with her eyes, it's like I woke up.

I saw me. My inner child who wanted nothing more than to be loved. And I realised at that moment that I had turned into my mum and all the women before her, unleashing generations of internalised misogyny, violence and suffering onto the one person I'd always vowed to protect.

I knew that I wanted better for my daughter. I knew that I wanted her to grow up free from my wounds, to be able to fully express herself, to love herself and know her worth and give her the freedom to live *her* life, not mine.

When I looked at my daughter, full of unconditional love, so pure and innocent, when I realised that her challenging behaviour was a mirror of me, I knew that I had to set myself free from my shadow.

The generational wounds had to stop with me so that I could leave a better legacy for my children.

Reader Notes:

Who you are *being*-not what you are doing -has the greatest impact on your children.

If you want to raise children who live as the fullest expression of themselves -physically, emotionally and spiritually including all the messy parts - then *you* need to be the change. *You* need to be that person.

It doesn't matter how cool, calm and conscious a parent you are *if* you're bypassing your shadow. The more you deny your shadow, the more power it has and the more reactive you are to it. And your children are the greatest reflection of your shadow and the greatest gift for your own awakening.

Be honest with yourself. Look beneath your triggers. Face your deepest, darkest, most uncomfortable truths. Feel all the feelings, no matter how uncomfortable. *Own* your darkness. Because stepping into your shadow is *the* source of your liberation. And by freeing yourself you heal the past and future generations too.

Author Bio:

Michelle Catanach is on a mission to end childism and violence against children and is passionate about alleviating depression and anxiety in our kids and teens. She helps children master their energy and emotions and be the leader of their life. She is also the founder of Uncaged Online, a creative agency for paradigm-shifters to reach the masses with their message through book publishing, web design, content creation and digital products.

Connect with Michelle:

Website: www.michellecatanach.co.uk &
www.uncaged.online
Instagram: @michelle_catanach

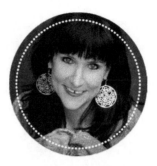

Breaking the Silence
By Anne Corazza

'Trauma is not what happens to us, but what we hold inside in the absence of an empathetic witness.' ~ *Peter A Levine*

I was 22 years old when I had my first real suicide attempt.

I had recently graduated from college and was working part-time at four different jobs. I worked seven days a week. I stayed as busy as possible because it was all I had ever known.

I just found out I had landed a full-time dream job, working for a state-wide youth development program. We empowered young people to make healthy choices free of alcohol, tobacco and other drugs by providing leadership training and peer-mentoring.

It was a massive undertaking, and I thought I was perfect for the job. You see, I was naive enough to believe that it was my mission in life to save the world from alcohol and drug abuse. I was convinced it was the number one problem in society. It caused child abuse, domestic violence, divorce, rape, adultery and wars. My childhood was a living hell due to alcohol, and I hated it with every fibre of my being. I had also been the victim of sexual assault by two different perpetrators and had decided that I would never, ever have sex. It was scary, nasty, evil and something I never wanted to be a part of ever again.

Despite my extreme views, I thought I could be a positive role model for teenagers to deter them from making unhealthy choices. As it turns out, I *was* perfect for the job, but not for the reasons I thought. I could not stop the abuse or save the world. But, I could relate to all the struggles and pain these young people were facing at home.

Alcohol abuse in their homes was the norm for many along with sexual abuse, violence, verbal abuse, emotional abuse, divorce and adultery. I knew exactly why she was failing history class or why he wouldn't look me in the eye; they were starving, sleep deprived, paranoid and had zero self-worth.

The lies.
The secrets.
The confusion.
The fear.
The shame.
It broke my heart!

I was good at the work I did, and the teens seemed to relate to me and look up to me as a big sister. It felt so good to know I was able to make a small difference in empowering these young people to believe in themselves and give them the confidence to influence their peers positively.

From the outside, I had a great life. Highly respected by my bosses, peers and community collaborators, I appeared happy and was doing a job I loved more than anything. Working late nights and many weekends, I couldn't have had any more passion for the work I did to help young people with the challenges I knew about first hand.

I also had a boyfriend at this time who I felt was a saint to be with me because he knew how damaged I was. I wanted so badly for someone to love me, but I was scared to get close to anyone. I honestly thought all men were sexually aggressive and wanted only one thing. But, my new boyfriend was different. He knew I was damaged goods but still wanted to be with me. He knew I was not able to have intercourse due to severe flashbacks and he would never force himself on me.

Sometimes we would be kissing, and suddenly I would get gut-wrenching flashbacks and freeze. All these memories would come rushing back. I could see the other guy; I could hear him, smell him, and still feel the welts on my skin. I was so frustrated because I felt safe with my boyfriend and enjoyed kissing him but would suddenly shut down. I would check out of my body, laying there limp as an empty shell.

My boyfriend was amazing. He was there for me one hundred percent and would just hold me or make me talk to him to bring me back to the room. He also knew things about my childhood. I started to share with him secrets that I'd never told anyone, such as self-harming since I was 14. I didn't know why I did it other than hating myself to my core. I was broken. Damaged. I could not look at myself in the mirror. I hated what I saw. I was ugly. I didn't know any other way to punish myself or to shred the pain and self-hatred.

I started having suicidal thoughts when I was about 16 years old. Throughout my college years, the thoughts became more and more frequent to the point that I was waking every single morning wishing I was dead. I put on a brave face, a fake smile and a mask. But, behind closed doors, I would be curled up in a ball in bed crying for hours.

So here I was, aged 22, waking up in the hospital with a tube down my throat. The first person I saw when I opened my eyes was the doctor. He leaned over my bed and said: 'Now aren't you glad you did not succeed?' I was horrified! My mind started to race, my insides burning. *Oh, my God, I am still here*, I thought to myself. Sheer panic rushed through my veins. *NO! Please NO! This can't be real. I hope I am dreaming.*

It was true. My attempt to end it all had failed. I burst into tears. It hurt to cry with the tube down my throat. My thoughts continued to spin out of control. *How the hell am I going to deal with the shame and embarrassment of others finding out that I have tried to end my life?* I couldn't even do this right. I wanted to escape my pathetic existence more than ever.

I knew that most people felt it was selfish to end one's life. But, I was convinced my boyfriend deserved someone better. I was a master people pleaser and usually considered everyone else's needs before my own. I knew it would profoundly affect the young people I was mentoring. What kind of message would that send to them? But, I had gotten to the point where none of that mattered anymore. I just couldn't be in this much pain any longer.

I was released after several days. I started seeing a therapist 2 or 3 times per week and attending Al-Anon meetings, but I still wanted to die. I would tell my therapist everything. It was insane as I was still working full-time on the program with the youth. I lived two lives, pouring everything into my job while secretly wishing that I was dead. I hated being me.

The Wounded Healer

Several years later I went to the gun store and tried to buy a gun; as it turns out, they have a three-day waiting period, so I left empty-handed. The next day I stormed to my therapist and told her what I'd done. Before I knew what was happening, she and her 300-pound muscular roommate were dragging me into her car, kicking and screaming.

I was taken to a lock-up facility and stripped of everything including the barrette in my hair for fear that I might harm myself. I was the only female. A man stood at a table talking to Jesus. Several other guys were playing cards. And one guy was rocking back and forth in the corner on the floor. This was all the confirmation I needed. *I am 100% bonafide crazy!* It reaffirmed every negative thought I had ever had about myself.

After three days, I moved to the women's centre which was full of 'crazy' women like me, all struggling with the same issues: depression, suicide, sexual abuse, physical abuse, drug abuse, etc. I was there for over a month, my outside therapist visiting every other day. I continued with therapy twice a week with her for another eight years. She was an angel in my life. I went to Al-Anon meetings for about 12 years followed by Codependents Anonymous for a further six years.

By age 29, I was finally able to look at myself in the mirror. This was after years of friends telling me over and over how beautiful I was. Before this, I would burst into tears every time I looked. I honestly thought I was the ugliest person on the planet.

After ten years working for the youth program and acknowledging that I was a workaholic, I stepped down, and instead trained as a Holistic Health Practitioner/Massage Therapist to create more balance in my life. It was at this time that I finally acknowledged that I had been a healer my entire life. I can sense intuitively what is going on in almost any environment. I can read other people, and I feel very deeply. I have been this way since I was a small child, doing whatever I could to heal the suffering and chaos in my own family. I often feel other people's pain including strangers so intensely that it makes me physically sick. But, this allows me the gift of deep empathy, compassion and an ability to help others heal.

I slowly pulled myself out of the rabbit hole, yet the memories would continue to creep back in. I wanted so badly to let go of the past, but the trauma felt trapped in every cell of my body.

Finding My Voice

My Dad was a workaholic, a drunk, a narcissist and a cheat with quite an angry streak. I was scared to death of him, spending hours hiding in the closet. My sister was also extremely angry and would beat the crap out of me regularly. I do not blame her. She learned it from our Dad; she did to me what was done to her. I remember when I was only seven years old visiting the library and reading about alcoholism. I was already trying to help others and desperately wanted to find a way to fix my family.

My Dad left when I was 11. He got up super early one Sunday morning, packed up all his things and walked out without saying goodbye. My Mom was devastated, spending the next month sitting out on the back patio getting drunk, smoking and not eating. She would cry all day every day, as did I. Despite everything, I missed him. But most importantly I was worried about my Mom and felt it was my responsibility to ease her pain. This began the start of my full-time role of care-giver as she slipped further and further into alcoholism.

My sister was 3.5 years older and dealt with things very differently. I was always trying to fix things while she remained in her room with her door closed, angry and isolated. Other times she would be yelling and physically taking her anger out on me. I learned humility from my sister, as I could not do anything right in her eyes. She felt it was her duty to correct my every word and let me know all day every day what I was doing wrong. I learned I was stupid, ugly, broken and defective. Since she was older, I felt guilty that she took the brunt of my Dad's temper. Perhaps I was the one thing she felt she could have power over.

I felt so very alone my entire childhood. I had no one, and I mean *no one*, to validate my experience. To the outside world we were the perfect, happy family yet the abuse and toxicity behind closed doors told a completely different story.

The abuse continued well into adulthood until I *finally* felt strong enough to find my voice, which only made things worse. The more I spoke my truth, the greater the backlash. I was accused of being weak, a liar, a fantasist. Of clinging to the past. Yet, as I see it, I am the only one courageous enough to do the work needed to truly heal.

My Secret Life

I continue to have challenges with Post Traumatic Stress Disorder; my health has been a challenge my entire life. First, severe asthma starting as an infant from dogs and cigarette smoke. I took steroids and a multitude of other medications regularly my whole childhood. Between the ages of 11 and 14, I was bitten numerous times by ticks as our backyard was a forest.

In my early 30's my health took a severe dive. I landed in the hospital with pancreatitis followed by strange bouts where the right side of my body would curl up. I would have tremors or paralysis. Sometimes it would last a few hours or a couple of days. I had ongoing blood in my urine, digestive issues, chronic pain, heart problems, cognitive challenges and ringing in my ears. I went to doctor after doctor, and none of them could piece it together. Eventually diagnosed with severe leaky gut and Fibromyalgia, no explanation for the neurological problems or the daily fluctuating fevers was given.

In 2007, I tested positive with Late-Stage Neurological Lyme Borreliosis with a multitude of co-infections, 30 years after the original tick bites. This is a blood disease that affects every system in your body causing damage to your bones, heart, brain, muscles, digestion, kidneys, hormones, nerves and of course your immune system. But, the hardest thing about having this disease is that scientific research is being suppressed causing most doctors to lack adequate education about it, and we are left to feel that our symptoms are all in our head.

I suffer from daily pain, fevers and seizures on the right side of my body where my muscles curl up. My diet is very limited. Most people have no idea what I experience on a daily basis because on the outside I look normal. Invisible Chronic Illness became another secret that I had to carry. It is painful when others tell us that we don't 'look' sick meanwhile we are ravaged with pain and the infections are eating us alive on the inside.

Lyme Disease is something I am working on accepting instead of fighting. Colds and the flu eventually go away. But when you have a chronic illness, one must learn to accept it. And, of course, I know it could always be much worse.

The pivotal moment for me was when I was bedridden for months on end, unable to function. I was too sick to work, and I could no longer hide behind being a do-aholic, the one thing that had always been my coping mechanism. After seven years of treatment and financially broke, I was barely surviving. I felt like a caged animal in this body, yet too tired to fight anymore.

It would have been easy to give up. But, I had lost three dear friends to suicide and promised myself I would be a voice for those who suffer in silence. I dreamed of finding a way out of my suffering so that I could help the masses and leave a powerful legacy behind.

So, I started to ask myself the tough questions. Why am I here? What is my purpose? I read every empowering book I could get my hands on. I watched inspiring YouTube videos like The Secret, Abraham Hicks, Tony Robbins, Danielle LaPorte and Oprah Winfrey. Personal development became my lifeline, helping me much more than therapy ever had. It was the medicine my soul was craving. I was hooked.

The Pursuit of Joy

I started to take baby steps to *love myself* by acknowledging my bravery and big heart. I practised being more conscious and present, letting go of beliefs that no longer served me. I started thinking about what my dreams might be. How did I want to feel? What were the things in my life that made me happy or brought me joy?

One of the most enlightening things I learned was that the main purpose of our life is to follow our heart and do what makes us happy, to pursue joy. *Really?* This seemed so foreign to me. *I have lived my entire life in survival, in fear,*

I thought. Even when I had a safe place to lay my head at night, I felt trapped in a sick body with financial worries. How the heck are you supposed to 'follow joy' when you are in survival mode? It seemed selfish.

After more reflection, I realised that I had experienced plenty of moments of joy in my life, I simply wasn't focusing on them. Yes, my life was hard, but the joy was there, buried beneath layers of depression and despair. I had kept a gratitude journal for years, and I was indeed grateful for many things, especially for incredible friends who were earth angels. One dear friend suggested writing down three things that made me happy at the end of each day. I discovered that, while I could write ten things I was grateful for, not one thing made me happy.

Over time this became easier. Seeing a hummingbird fly. Hugging a friend. Spending time in nature. Watching a comedy. Reading. But, my biggest discovery has been creative expression. I love to dance as it has allowed me to shut down my brain and be present. I also discovered I have a deep passion for writing, art and I crave solitude in nature.

My new purpose in life is to do more things that make me happy and to have fun! I am now on a quest to focus on the joy in life. To make my dreams come true. It is a conscious spiritual practice. I listen to when things raise my vibration and take it as a sign to allow more of it into my life.

I am now rewriting my story. It's no longer about a broken-hearted disaster, but a self-love, chase your dreams kinda story. We all have the power to rewrite our story, to find the bliss in each moment, to become the heroine of our own life.

Today, I love myself, with all my perfectly, imperfect parts. My life still has its challenges. But, today I choose to no longer be a victim in silence. I needed to go back and remember who I was before I experienced any trauma. I am here to *be love*, that is what I truly came here to do. I am here to grow, evolve and help others on their journey. I have learned that I am a very sensitive person in a very messy world. I am a spiritual being, having a human experience. We all have challenges. I am not broken. I am a warrior.

It was through the writing of my life story that I have experienced my greatest growth. It has given me a platform to share my truth. It has been one of the scariest things I have ever done, but keeping silent to the shame just perpetuates the cycle of denial. It only gives consent to my own or others unacceptable behaviour in my life. I no longer choose to be bound by secrets. As I shine light on my shadow, the darkness slowly fades away.

For me, in the end, love, truth and bravery are all that matter. We must be there for one another. We need to be the light for those who suffer in silence. But first we must learn to love ourselves; love is what our souls are meant to do.

I have learned that sharing our stories can help us to heal. It helps us rise above the pain and make more conscious, clear choices. Today I say yes to life with all its pain, beauty, sorrow and bliss. Today, I choose to turn my mess into my message.

By being unapologetically *you*, speaking *your* truth, loving *all* of you, and choosing *joy* in all that you do you will energetically attract those who are meant to cross your path. New passions and career paths will naturally present themselves. By doing what you love and following the joy in your heart, you will naturally help others along the way.

So, now I selfishly put my oxygen mask on first, and it is amazing how much lighter I feel. How much more free I am becoming. It is so liberating to choose joy.

Reader Notes:

Joy is your internal guidance system. And if it isn't a hell yes, then it is a definite no. Find the things that make you joyful.

Creative self-expression is a beautiful way to connect with your true essence, express how you feel, allow energy to move, experience joy and release what may be troubling you. How can you allow yourself to *play* today?

Create a vision board of words, images and ideas that your heart deeply desires.

At the end of each day, list three things that made you happy today. Keep them on your phone, in your art journal or in a jar by your bed. Revisit them often. By the end of the year, you will have a beautiful list of some amazing memories to bring a smile to your face.

Author Bio:

Anne Corazza aka The Uncaged Artist is an Author, Speaker, Mixed-Media Artist, Intuitive Healer, Life Coach, Self-Love Catalyst, Chief Happiness Officer, BeREAL Advocate and Transformational Leader who is passionate about helping those who suffer in silence to find their voice, share their story, release shame and set themselves free through creative expression. Anne inspires her clients to lead a more conscious, peaceful, happy life using the power of art as medicine.

Anne is a true testament to rising above life's challenges by finding the courage to shine a light on one's darkness and learning to find inspiration and joy in each day. From no longer seeing a purpose to live, ravaged with a lifetime of pain and suffering in silence, Anne is now on a mission to reach the masses with her message and help lost souls find themselves again.

Connect with Anne:

Website: www.TheUncagedArtist.com
FB: www.facebook.com/TheUncagedArtist
Instagram: @theuncagedartist

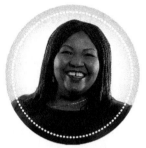

Breaking the Mould
By Ruth Oshikanlu

'Break the mould! Have the biggest vision you can! If you can't dream it, it cannot occur!' ~ Judy Baca

I had to look up the word 'badass' in the dictionary, as it's not a word that I would have used to describe myself. The dictionary defined badass as 'a tough, uncompromising or intimidating person'. Oh, so I am a badass then! I am a non-conformist, and I love it! I believe I was born free, and my mission in life is to remain so.

So how did I become a badass?

I believe I was born a badass. My struggle has been to remain this way. Here's my story.

Rough Ruth (Age 0-10)

I was born the eldest and only daughter of three children to Nigerian parents, who were very loving. I came from a strong line of matriarchs; my great-grandmother, grandmother and mum being very strong-willed and feisty women, so it was easy for me to follow in their footsteps. This was fine at home. However, before long, I realised that being a strong-willed girl who did not conform to societal expectations was going to pose a problem.

Nigeria is a patriarchal country where men and women have clearly defined roles with men having more power and being decision-makers, and women expected to be subservient and not challenge decisions made by men. For instance, polygamy is a common practice, and a married man could decide to take another wife, and his first wife had no right to question this decision. If she did not like his decision, she was free to leave. If she had children, she could not take her children with her, as the children bear her husband's name, and as such, belonged to him.

This was my grandmother's story. Despite bearing five children for my grandfather, he decided to marry another woman. But my grandmother was not going to share a husband. Hence, she left and later set up her own business and has been independent ever since.

As a young child, I admired my grandmother's free spirit and wanted so much to be like her. Being raised around two brothers, they were free to do so much, like climbing trees and playing with rubber tyres. I wanted to do the same too. I was also quite competitive. If my brothers climbed a tree, I felt compelled to prove I could do the same. Unfortunately, I was often wearing a skirt or dress which made it more difficult. This was how I developed a preference for wearing trousers.

I also detested having my hair in plaits and asked my parents to cut my hair whenever my brothers had their hair cut.

I disliked the roles assigned to girls such as helping with cooking and cleaning and preferred to play with my brothers. I often thought: If we are all going to eat, why don't we all have to cook? Why am I the only one cooking and cleaning? Fortunately, my parents were liberal and respected my views. However, I struggled outside the home. When I played with friends and cousins, I was often rough and heavy-handed. They refused to play with me, complaining that I played like a boy and so I earned the name 'Rough Ruth!'

Rebellious Ruth (Age 11-20)

I was a very bright child, and my parents saw my potential and fostered its development. By age nine, I was in one of the best girls' schools in Nigeria, Queen's College, Lagos. I was a big kid and quite feisty, and so it did not take me long to settle into school and find my place. I loved being in school and enjoyed learning which was quite competitive. I also enjoyed standing up for people who were bullied. I went through puberty quite early, and although I was young, people often thought that I was much older as I was fully developed and was tall with big feet. I often struggled with having conversations with my peers, as they usually wanted to talk about boys.

At home, I struggled with my mum, especially in my teens as I was mouthy and always wanted to have the last word. When she asked me to do something at home, I would ask for the rationale. This was deemed rude in our culture. Adults, especially parents, had every right to tell you what to do and you had no right to question them. My catchphrase in this period was often: 'This is not fair!' to which I would get the response: 'Life is not fair!' My mission was to exasperate my mum, and I am very sure I did, although this did not make life easy for me. Her purpose was to endeavour to reign me, like a wild horse.

My father, realising that I was strong-willed, used reverse-psychology with me. If he wanted me to go right, he would ask me to go left, knowing that I would do the opposite. That way, he got me to do what he wanted without me realising it. It was win-win. As such, I had no friction with my father. He doted on me. All I had to do was ensure that I had excellent grades, and he pushed me to be the best I could be. He wanted me to study medicine, and for a while I went along with his plan. However, in my late teens, I decided that this was my father's dream and not mine and left Nigeria for England.

Upon arriving in England, I knew I was going to continue my education but was unsure what to study. Although my father wanted me to train as a doctor, I chose not to, which disappointed him greatly. After trying out a few courses, I decided to qualify as a nurse, which my father considered a waste of my talent. I completed my nurse training and still could not determine what area of nursing to specialise in. One day, while working in the accident and emergency department, I saw a baby being born and knew instantly that I wanted to become a midwife.

Radical Ruth (age 20-30)

I thoroughly enjoyed my midwifery training and felt being 'with woman' (meaning of the word *midwife*) in pregnancy, childbirth and after the birth of the baby was my life's purpose. However, I hated how medicalised childbirth was. As a newly qualified midwife, I remember caring for a woman in labour. She was having regular contractions and coping with labour pains. And so was her unborn baby. Then an obstetrician came to review her and deemed her as progressing 'slowly', according to policy. Her labour was augmented (sped up) with drugs. Within an hour, she was no longer coping, and her baby's heart rate dropped, and she had to be rushed to theatre for an emergency Caesarean. After her operation, she thanked the obstetrician for saving her baby's life. I was livid! I believed that this was a created and easily-avoided problem. If the woman was left to labour at her pace, both mother and baby would have coped with labour and avoided an operation.

I immediately decided that I was not going to be a part of medicalised childbirth and skilled myself up to be able to support women who preferred to deliver their babies at home. I joined The Association of Radical Midwives, training in active birth methods and water births. I made it my mission to enable women to trust their bodies and birth their babies *their* way.

I thoroughly enjoyed being a community midwife. However, after a couple of years, I got burnt out as the role was quite demanding. There were days I would spend eighteen hours, supporting a woman labouring at home, meaning that I had little time for myself outside of work. It was then I had the realisation that I was attracted to working with vulnerable groups of clients. I trained to become a HIV specialist midwife, and started supporting HIV-positive pregnant women. I thoroughly enjoyed this role as I got to form deep relationships with clients, advocate for them and empower them.

But one of my desires was to leave a legacy in the nursing and midwifery profession. I also wanted to do something positive in Africa. I decided to apply to Médicins Sans Frontières (a non-government organisation) who recommended that I acquire a Diploma in Tropical Nursing (DTN) to work for them. It was while doing the DTN course that I became pregnant, aged 30 years.

Resilient Ruth (Age 30-40)

Upon finding out I was pregnant, being a go-getter and a planner, I drew up what I thought was the perfect pregnancy plan and my home birth. I decided to move house as I felt that my flat was not ideal to raise a baby. I completed the DTN course, but halfway through my pregnancy, at a routine scan, it was discovered that I was in premature labour and my baby was on his way out. I had to be rushed to theatre for an emergency cervical stitch and was hospitalised for the rest of pregnancy. It was the most emotionally challenging period of my life as, although I knew what was happening to me, I did not know how to manage myself. I was also in denial. My life had been full of stress as I was trying to do so many stressful things while growing my baby. Being a free spirit, I struggled very much with being hospitalised and challenged every decision the doctors made. But I also recognised that despite not liking hospitals, it was the best place for my unborn baby and me. I also felt immense guilt. I had not made time for my baby in pregnancy. I cried so much for my unborn son to forgive me and promised him that I would make him a priority. I connected with him, decided to name him and pleaded with him to stay inside of me. As I was in a room by myself, and often the only company I had, I talked with him every minute I was awake. I played music to him and involved him in everything I did. It was lovely to see our relationship blossom as he responded to my communication by moving in my belly.

Unfortunately, due to pre-eclampsia in pregnancy and very high blood pressure, he had to be born prematurely. I told my unborn baby it was time to be born and he responded. It was a very long labour as he had managed to get himself tangled and had the cord tightly around his neck. Towards the end of labour, when the obstetrician reviewed me and stated that he was going to give me an hour to push, I pleaded with Joshua, declaring how much I wanted to deliver him naturally. It was so lovely how he responded by turning, just enough to untangle him slightly and within thirty minutes, he was born. Despite a few days of separation when he was admitted to the neonatal intensive care unit, we were eventually reunited and discharged home.

Unfortunately, a casualty of my long hospitalisation in pregnancy was my relationship with Joshua's father. While hospitalised, he had tried to care for Joshua and me while holding a job. But nothing he did was to my satisfaction. I felt I had been cheated. All the time I thought: 'We made the baby. You're free! I'm stuck in hospital!' And I took it out on him. By the time I had Joshua, I had already decided that I would raise him alone.

Returning home to an empty house was very scary. I was happy to be free. But I was terrified. I had been in a hospital for so long that I think I had become institutionalised. I was also paranoid and heard the sounds of machines in the night. The realisation of the weighty responsibility of parenting hit me. But my Joshua was such a lovely and contented baby. He was a delight to care for. And as soon as he started smiling, he never stopped.

I took a year out from work to raise him and thoroughly enjoyed it. When my year out was up, I started my health visitor training, inspired by the professional support my health visitors had provided in parenting Joshua. Upon qualifying as a health visitor, I took a specialist role in supporting pregnant teenagers and teenage parents. I loved the position and the difference I was making to marginalised groups. I guess that I too, as a single parent, was now deemed to be a marginalised group. Although I was happy as a single parent, I soon recognised that culturally, it was not acceptable. My parents and siblings were very supportive. But often, friends and extended family questioned if I was going to continue without a husband. I was made to feel like I was not complete without a man in my life.

It was then that I became even more determined to prove that single parents are not less than, but can achieve just the same as two-parent families. At the same time, I was having problems with my manager at work. I decided to leave the NHS to train as a life coach. After obtaining my coaching qualification, I trained in neuro-linguistic programming and other therapies such as cognitive behavioural therapy and set up a coaching consultancy. I focused on supporting professionals to be happy and productive at work. However, I missed working with women.

I decided to pen my first book *Tune In To Your Baby: Because Babies Don't Come with An Instructional Manual* as a way of sharing my professional and personal insights about pregnancy and the first few years of life. The aim of the book was to encourage parents to connect with their babies from conception and develop a relationship with them. I believed that was the reason I did not lose Joshua in pregnancy and wanted to support other women to do the same too.

Real Ruth (age 40)

Although I had achieved so much in my career and as a single parent, I felt I had not always been as authentic as I could have been. There were times I had kept quiet despite having objections. There were times I had not challenged the status quo. There were times I had not allowed myself to be seen and heard. If I was to be real, I would have to be more visible and audible. I started writing for publications and being more visible on social media. I put myself forward for projects that I was passionate about such as contributing to government policy on Female Genital Mutilation.

Then I completed my Masters degree in parental-foetal attachment and how midwives and health visitors can promote it. I have since launched a service *Pregnancy without Fear* to support women (and their partners) who have had assisted conception or recurrent miscarriage and are pregnant and scared. I love helping these women as it reminds me of how I was and how I wished I'd had someone like me to support me.

Looking back my life has been one of defying expectations. Society sets expectations, demands things of us, mainly as girls and women. We're handed a mould to which we're expected to conform. My life has been one of breaking the mould and defying all expectations. My mission is to be the woman I wished I had when I needed a woman most. If I am to continue towards my purpose, then I must not be squeezed into a box. I must shape myself and continue to defy expectations that others have set for me. For now, I am enjoying being an authentic soul and doing things my way! I urge you to do the same too.

Reader Notes:

The only time you should ever look back, is to see how far you have come.

As a nurse, I had the privilege of looking after many people as they were dying. Their main regrets they had were their unfulfilled dreams that were passing away with them and the relationships they never mended whilst they could. This has been a motivating factor for me to living a fulfilled life spending time with those that truly matter to me. I know how I want to feel as I am dying. I know the legacy I want to live behind.

Can you say the same?

Pause now and think about where you would like to be at the end of your life.
How do you want to feel?

What would you want to be said about you?

We all plan to live a long life. But there are no guarantees. I have nursed many that died prematurely. I've also learned that it's not how long you live but the difference you make when you are alive.

In order to live a fulfilled life, I have looked back in life to see how far I have come and tried to summarise my life in decades with words starting with the letter R for Ruth.

Why not try the same exercise. It will enable you to gauge your progress and shape the time you have left.

Author Bio:

Ruth Oshikanlu aka The Serene and Soulful Mama's Coach, is a nationally recognised expert nurse, midwife, health visitor and parenting expert. Ruth is passionate about parenting believing that good enough parenting is the best gift a parent can give to a child. She is drawn to working with marginalised communities and has been involved with delivering numerous projects to meet the needs of vulnerable and socially excluded groups including supporting HIV positive pregnant women and new mums; pregnant teenagers and teenage parents; and women affected by Female Genital Mutilation.

Being a single parent and part of a marginalised group in society, Ruth wants to be a role model for other single parents. She believes that ordinary people can achieve extraordinary things. She is willing to put her ahead above the parapet, challenging the status quo to improve client experience and the quality of care provided.

Ruth is the author of *Tune In To Your Baby: Because Babies Don't Come with An Instruction Manual* and creator of Tune In To Your Baby™ - a holistic parenting programme that enables pregnant women and new mothers develop secure attachments with their babies from the womb. To date, she has supported thousands of women and babies in pregnancy, labour and childbirth, the postnatal period through to toddlerhood. Her mission is to enable as many women as she can to enjoy parenting without sacrificing their own personal needs.

Ruth is The Pregnancy Mindset Expert and recently launched a private practice in London's Harley Street. She equips pregnant women who have had assisted conception or experienced previous pregnancy loss with the tools to manage anxiety, fear and stress so that they can remain pregnant, bond with their baby before birth, promoting maternal and infant mental health. She is a regular columnist and has published several feature articles in numerous national nursing and healthcare journals.

She is tenacious and has developed resilience through her experiences and encourages others to do the same. In her spare time, she mentors and coaches young girls with low self-esteem.

Ruth is a Queen's Nurse, Fellow of The Institute of Health Visiting and Royal College of Nursing. She is a recipient of several national clinical and business awards.

Connect with Ruth:

Website: www.tuneintoyourbaby.com
Twitter: @RuthOshikanlu
Instagram: @ruthoshikanlu
LinkedIn: Ruth Oshikanlu
Facebook: Tune In To Your Baby

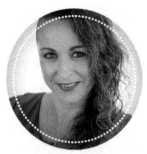

From Broken to Badass
By Laura Francis

'Whatever you hold in your mind on a consistent basis is exactly what you will experience in your life'
~ Tony Robbins

'So does that mean that I can smack you in the face now?'

Seriously. That's what I asked him. And he said 'Yes'. So I did.

Instantly that question became one of the worst questions I have ever asked. And what happened next defined me.

Because then, at that very moment, everything changed for me. My world exploded into a nightmare that I should have been able to predict but I never honestly thought was possible.

But this wasn't a dream.

This was my reality.
This is what I was living
This was what I was feeling.

Everything that I thought was... wasn't.

The situation in my parents' house was out of control. That's how it was with my family. It was impossible to know from one minute to the next what would happen. Which I guess is perfectly normal. Understandable even. Because we cannot predict what will happen in the future. We can only imagine.

But things were almost always volatile. Palpable. Ready to explode. Well, maybe not things but people.

If it wasn't my mother screaming venomous, degrading abuse at my siblings and me, it was one of my siblings doing it. Or else it was full-blown war. And I don't mean the type that involves soldiers and guns but domestic violence.... child abuse was the name of the game in that household.

I get it though.

And it took me a long time to understand. But now I do. It's all they knew. They weren't able to do things any different. They became broken - all of them - within the first few years of their lives. Their behaviour was cyclic.

If I didn't already feel unwanted and broken and like I couldn't trust a single person in the world, this day proved that to me once and for all.

The Day That Changed My Life

I was 16. It was morning. I was all but ready to head off to school.

A short while earlier one of my sisters had called him a bastard. He was convinced it was me, and after berating and abusing me for it, my father smacked me across the face.

I was so upset and scared shitless.

But I was confident that I could show him, that I could persuade him, that I could prove to him that I hadn't done that 'thing' that I was blamed for. Abused for. That I'd been hit for.

And I did.

You'd think I'd have been happy with that. But no. I wanted to take things one step further. I wanted him to feel what I felt. Just a little bit.

So when I asked that dreaded questions, and he said yes... fearfully, trying to keep the conversation light... trying to make light of an awful situation... trying to trust that everything would be alright...

I did it.
I hit him.

I smacked my father in the face.

It was just a tap really because I was terrified to unleash the real depth of my pain, my heartache, and frustration. And as soon as I did it I wished that I hadn't.

You see, that smack I gave my father was like a red flag to a bull.

It all happened so fast I had no time to become aware of what was happening or avoid it. In what felt like nanoseconds he launched at me and punched me so hard in the face, the head, the body, *everywhere.*

If I thought I was scared or terrified before, I was wrong. Because in the few minutes that this particular beating lasted I honestly thought I was going to die.

Don't get me wrong, this was not the first time. But it was by far the worst time. It felt like it would never end.

We were the only ones at home at this time. Just the two of us.

My father pushed me. He punched me. He kicked me all over the kitchen. I had nowhere to turn. There was no-one to help me. No-one to protect me.

The person who I trusted to do that (up until this moment) was busily beating me like I was a grown man in a pub brawl instead of loving, honouring, respecting and looking out for me as fathers are supposed to do.

My head was reeling. My heart was racing.

I didn't know what to do or how to escape. I was trapped. Like a caged animal.

And then, just as I thought things couldn't possibly get any worse, it happened.

He had me backed into a corner, literally a dishwasher space, and I was curled up into the tightest ball, the tightest foetal position I could curl myself up into, with no way out.

And for what seemed like an eternity my father continued to kick and punch me.

This man that I had trusted.
This man that I had looked up to.
This man that I had admired.
This man that I had loved.
This man that I thought loved me.
This man that I had adored.

Showed me the truth of what he was. Of who he was. Of his love and respect for me.

I don't know how long the beating lasted, maybe 5 or 10 minutes, but at some point, he stopped. His rage ended. He cooled down and walked out of the house.

I lay there, curled up tight. Afraid to move or make a noise.

And then once I felt it was safe to do so, I prised myself out of that dishwasher space and raced to my bedroom where I collected my school bag and ran from the house.

But where could I go?

I couldn't think clearly. But I knew I couldn't go to the hospital because if I did the police would likely be called, and my father might get arrested, and despite everything, I couldn't let that happen.

I had to protect him. And I had to protect myself from getting another beating like the one I'd just received.

So I rode my bike to my sister's house about 15 minutes away.

Blood streamed down my face. My eyes were swollen. Lumps, bumps and bruises already showed on my tender skin. My head. My face. My ribs. My back. All were aching beyond belief.

As I rode, things became clearer. And I decided that from here on in I would trust no-one.

That remained my truth for many, many years. And I proved it to be right, time and time again.

I couldn't trust my family - my mother or my father.
I couldn't trust my sisters nor my brothers.
I couldn't trust my lovers or my friends.
I put up an invisible wall, so big and robust that no-one could get through, over or around. So that I felt protected. Safe.

And on the rare occasion that I let someone in, that I allowed them to get into my heart... that person would always prove me right again.

But what really happened, what I failed to realise, what I couldn't see, what I didn't understand, is that in refusing to allow myself to trust anyone I was also refusing to trust myself.

I taught myself to not trust my judgement.
I taught myself to not trust my decisions.
I taught myself to not trust my actions.

Of course, I didn't know that; I didn't become aware of that until my late 30's. I had no idea of the truth of it.

Now though, when I reflect back on my life I can see with crystal clarity where, when and how this impacted me in so many ways. How it affected my life and the lives of those around me. Close to me.

In my relationships.
In my work.
In my business.

Living in Denial

It took a long time to work through the reality of the ripple effect of that incident. To understand how to move through it. Past it.

I'd suppressed that emotional and mental pain, suffering, anguish and loneliness for so long that when it came time to go within and unlock the truth behind my lack of trust, I honestly struggled to unearth it.

I'd blocked it out for so long, pretending that I'd dealt with all of the shit that came with it. But in reality, I was living in denial. And living in denial doesn't serve us. It is, in fact, extremely toxic.

Living in denial and refusing to accept, acknowledge and own the truth of those experiences, we're left small. It forces us to live less of a life than we were born to live. It holds us in a place of pain and suffering, of not-enoughness, of unhappiness. Of being the victim.

Breaking the Chains

Here's the thing.

Those things that our parents do to us.
Those things that those we trust do to us.

They shape us.

But.

Ultimately, we get to choose how. We get to decide whether that stuff shapes us in negative or in positive ways. In ways that do not or in ways that do serve us.

And if we are not happy with the choice we have made, at any time, anytime at all, we get to choose again.

So I did.

We can choose to take the path of self-pity and victim-stance. Allowing those experiences to become our stories that we carry throughout our entire lives, and letting them impact us in unlimited ways. Giving the past permission to keep us stuck in our own stuckness, with feelings of sadness, lovelessness, loneliness, distrust.

Constantly disempowered.
Always not enough.
Blaming past situations and circumstances.

Or.

We can choose to rise above all of that shit, to take the valuable lessons that lie within those experiences and use those to create goodness in the world. In ourselves. In our lives. And in the lives of others. We can experience lives filled with happiness, joy, and freedom. Of being enough. Of loving ourselves wholly, unapologetically and unconditionally. And trusting in the infinite power that is the self that lies within you.

Knowing that you are supported.
That you are powerful.
That you are purposeful.
That you are happiness.

That loving and trusting yourself is all that you will ever need.

Reader Notes:

Journal Prompts:

I encourage you to dig really deep into the questions below; to go far below the initial surface level answers/responses that come up for you. So you get to experience maximum expansion and permanent transformation it is important that you give yourself permission to fully speak your truth; to go where you've previously been too afraid to go. And to not be afraid of your truth.

Remember.

No-one else needs to see your answers.

This is a purely selfish act *(in a really awesome way)* - for the greater good of **you**!

If you find that you're stuck and unable to write, walk away from your journal and take 3 deep breaths - in / out... in / out... in / out.

Then pick up your pen and let the stream of consciousness (writing organically without thought and filters) flow through you.

1. Where in my life am I still showing up as that scared little girl?
   What am I afraid of?
   How is this impacting my relationships right now?
   What can I do right now to change that?

2. Where in my life do I not allow myself to speak my truth for fear of retribution?
   How do I see that this fear is serving or protecting me?
   What is the worst thing that could happen if I were to choose to release that fear?
   What would my life look, feel and be if I were to choose to release that fear?

3. How is this my lack of trust in my own judgement, decisions and actions affecting me in my business and life right now?

   How is this lack of trust in myself serving me right now?

   What's the worst thing that would happen if I were to trust?

   Is this true?

4. What beliefs do I currently have around self-trust? Dig deep and list them out.

   If I were to allow myself to fully trust in my own judgement, decisions and actions, what would I be doing differently now?

   Who would I be showing up as?

   How would I be showing up?

   If I were showing up as this person, what belief systems would I have around

   self-trust? Dig deep into this and list them out.

Affirmations:

Repeat the following affirmations multiple times throughout the day, every day, for 30 days:

It is ok for me to trust myself unconditionally.

It is safe for me to trust in my own judgements, decisions and actions.

It is easy for me to trust myself to make judgements, decisions and to take actions that serve my higher self and for the higher good.

I trust myself fully every day. My judgements are sound, I am a brilliant decision maker and I take fast and decisive action while honouring my truth and living my life as the highest version of myself.

I release all fear of trusting myself and the burden of that to the Universe for it to work it's magic.

Write them.
Speak them.
Journal them.
Meditate on them.

Author Bio:

Since she was just 15 years old, Laura Francis has been studying personal development and business.

She thrives on inspiring women entrepreneurs tap into their hidden potential and align with their higher selves. Her high impact, make-it-happen strategies help you remove the mindset blocks stopping you from creating more leverage, money and freedom in your business and life.

Laura shows you how to shine your light on the world authentically, relentlessly and unapologetically by awakening your hidden genius and tapping into your core truth and souls purpose. Her transformative methods make doing the internal and external work, showing up, speaking your truth and attracting 'hell yes' soul-level clients a breeze.

Laura helps you own your truth, your desires and your passion and empowers you to show up, speak up and massively impact the world with your message and your purpose. Inspiring you to unleash the multi-6-figure mindset within so you can blow your results and your income out of the water.

Laura's here to help you to rise. To claim what's yours, including your crown and your throne so you can live the life you desire while being the Queen you were born to be. Charging what you're worth, leveraging your time and your profits selling low-high end digital courses and high-ticket VIP programs and events.

And of course, that means creating the multiple 6-figure online empire of your dreams. Because anything less is... well... it's non-negotiable.

Connect with Laura:

Website: www.laurafrancis.com.au
Facebook: www.facebook.com/iamlaurafrancis
Facebook Group: www.facebook.com/groups/365badass
Instagram: @laura_franciskam
Twitter: @LauraFrancisKAM

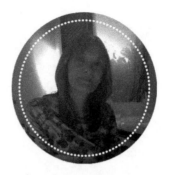

Indestructible Soul
By Alison Chan Lung

'I remember everything but forgive anyway.' ~ Erica Jong

Tick-tock. Tick-tock. The sound of the clock. The tick-tock seemed to resound around the silent, airless room. The door was locked. Curtains were drawn. Someone was standing over me. Hitting me. Punches reigned down onto my back. I lay face down on the floor.

I had gone to see a hypnotherapist because I couldn't sleep. I seemed to have permanent insomnia. It took me over an hour to drop off and then I would suddenly wake up and lay there for hours. It was affecting me and especially my work. Just as I was meant to be getting up for work, I'd fall into a deep sleep. Then I'd have to wake up and rush to get ready. Invariably I'd be late.

The hypnotherapist was a middle-aged man, and his voice was quite soothing. I wasn't sure if I could be hypnotised because my mind always seemed to be racing. But I drifted under with his words until all I could hear was the tick-tock. Tick-tock. Tick-tock. The sound of the clock. There was an actual clock in the room that was ticking quite loudly but as I went under it was another clock I heard.

Oh my God. I was back in that room. That silent, airless room. It was early 1977. I was 16. It had started as a silly flirtation by letter. Well, when I say letter I mean scrawled messages on school notebook paper. He was an acquaintance of my best friend and friend of her boyfriend. She would pass my notes onto him and he in return would send one back. It sounds pretty teenage now, and it was. I would sign my notes 'Juicy Lucy' who was a character in a film.

The notes went back and forth. It was something to do during a boring double session of history. He was older and seemed worldly wise. It was meant to be humorous banter and a bit of fun. I didn't have a boyfriend at the time, and my friend was spending a lot of time with her boyfriend in London where he lived. We lived in Pinner which was as exciting to us as having nothing to do and nowhere to go.

We'd outgrown suburbia with the twitching of the net curtains and the 2.4 families. My friend and I felt like we were the outcasts, the outsiders, the outliers.

We were drawn to each other. I was from an Irish mother and Chinese father which was unusual back then. She was into David Bowie and went through a phase where she liked to be called Ziggy. I was bullied at primary school for being different. We were bored of living in what seemed like a goldfish bowl. Swimming around and around with nowhere to go. It's no surprise that later that year we both got into punk and did our bit to fight against racism, fascism and misogyny.

An Invitation

When he phoned me to invite me to a party at his one weekend, I accepted the invitation without too much hesitation. Some fun, some excitement at last. He said that my friend's boyfriend would be there and mentioned some other people I knew. My friend was away on a school trip in France. It was to start in the daytime on Sunday. He said he would meet me at the station. He lived in Belsize Park. I told my Mum, and she seemed okay about it. She'd met my friend's boyfriend and knew him to be an upstanding chap (who later went on to become a successful TV producer).

We met at the station and walked back to his flat. We had met briefly before, but I guess this was the first time we had a chance to chat properly. I was slightly attracted to him but not overly. The notes we had written were probably a bit like the emails or messages people send on dating sites or Tinder these days. There's an element of fantasy because you don't know the person. I knew he had a flatmate and he said other guests would be arriving soon. For some reason, I had imagined there would be people already there.

The weather was cold, not yet Spring-like, and I hadn't really dressed for a party. I wore a long brown suede coat that belonged to my sister and even had a brown leather handbag of hers that was way too old for a 16-year-old. I looked more like 25. Not so much Juicy Lucy as Sophisticated Suzie.

When we walked into his flat, the first thing that struck me was that it was empty. He reassured me that people would be coming soon, so I sat down. He went to get a drink, and I was drawn to a box on the table. I don't know why but I looked inside and saw what looked like bones. Chicken bones possibly. I got a creepy feeling, and when he came back in, I asked about his flatmate. He looked down and said that he had tragically thrown himself under a train on the Paris metro. I didn't have a good feeling at all. He came and sat next to me.

He tried to kiss me. I kissed him back but knew straight away that I didn't feel anything for him. In fact, I felt repulsed by him. It was in that moment that my silly teenage infatuation crumbled into nothing. I had no feeling for him at all. I pulled away, and he tried to kiss me more. Close up all I could see were the large moles on his face and his cold blue eyes. I didn't want to lead him on any further and made it as clear as I could that I wouldn't sleep with him. I tried to get up, and he pulled me back down. He had a strange look on his face. My heart started to beat very fast. I asked when the others were coming and he said, 'they're not'.

Trapped

He got up and locked the door. He was stronger than me, and I knew I couldn't get out easily. All I could think was how to escape. I knew somewhere deep in me that I had to stay calm and somehow reason with him. I decided to appeal to his good nature. I still believed that he had one. But he had gone into a rant. The gist of it was something to do with his mother. Yes, the mother always gets blamed. I tried to be empathetic and to console him in some way. For a moment he physically backed away from me. I thought *this is my chance*. I tried to escape.

He, however, had other plans. He wanted to play a game. As soon as he said it I knew it would be a game I couldn't win.

He drew the curtains. Outside the sun had come out and it was still only mid-afternoon. I knew the world continued to exist outside this room and that I could still be a part of it. I kept thinking that I could get out of there somehow. That kept me going. We played his game. When I tell you the game, you'll shake your head in disbelief. It was a game of guess the number he was thinking. There was no way I could ever win.

I wanted to scream but knew I wouldn't be heard. The walls were very thick, and his flatmate was dead. Instead, I went silent. A voice inside me told me to stay very calm. Call it wisdom or intuition; it said to me *you will get through this*. But I felt like a little brown rabbit. And yet I knew that in my stillness I had some power. I can't explain it but I think it helped me somehow.

Of course, I couldn't guess any of the numbers in his head. I still tried to reason with him and let him know that my parents were expecting me back home. When I got the answers wrong he didn't act immediately, but eventually he got this cold, calculating look in his eyes. He pushed me down onto the floor and punched my back. It seemed like ages, and that's when I heard the tick-tock of the clock. The tick-tock was blocking out the sound of him hitting me and any noise I made. But like the little brown rabbit, I froze, and the adrenalin flooded my body, ensuring that I didn't feel the pain.

I was in shock. All I could think was that a decent person wouldn't treat a dog like this let alone a human being. He was careful not to hit my face or parts of me where the marks would show. Tick-tock. Tick-tock. And then it stopped. He let me get up. He let me go. But just to make sure, he escorted me to the station, my arm held tightly behind my back as he pushed me down the street. I suppose he didn't want me running to the nearest police station. I didn't care because now I could breathe in fresh air and any minute I'd be on that tube going home. I was free.

Coming Home

The tears came on the tube journey home. The next few days were awful. I didn't tell my Mum what happened, but maybe she sensed something. I woke up the following morning aching terribly. In fact, I was so severely bruised that I could hardly get out of bed. Walking hurt. I didn't go to school for a couple of days. I blamed myself for what had happened to me. I felt ashamed. I didn't tell anyone for a while, and I didn't report it. If I have any regrets in life that is one of them. But I can now see that I innocently got caught up in my own fearful thinking.

One positive thing to come out of this was that I turned to books. I'd always loved reading, and now I read anything by feminist authors or about women's empowerment. I read Marilyn French, Simone de Beauvoir, Germaine Greer, the

Shere Hite Report and Fear of Flying by Erica Jong. I wasn't going to let what happened to me stop me from doing what I wanted to do. I didn't want to be suspicious and untrusting of men and to have to suppress my sexuality or not be able to say no. When I told my best friend and my new lovely boyfriend what happened, I felt a sense of relief. At times I would feel incredibly angry. At other times I would come home to a peaceful feeling.

The hypnotherapist brought me back around. I opened my eyes and looked around the room. I was back in 1990. I started to sleep a bit better. Then a strange thing happened. I was looking at the photos of my best friend's recent wedding reception, and I had a sudden flashback to the happy day. I started sifting through the pictures thinking *oh my God, was that him?* I couldn't find photographic evidence but remembered talking to this man. It couldn't have been him, surely. He had come up to me at the wedding and spoke about his relationship with a Japanese woman.

I'd had a slight feeling of unease when he was talking to me yet couldn't pinpoint why. He must have known it was me. But now I was all grown up with my (then) husband standing nearby. I wasn't aware that it was him and afterwards, when my friend confirmed that it was, I felt angry. She said he had just turned up at the reception and she didn't know that he would come.

For a moment I remembered everything, but forgave anyway.

Reader Notes:

We are more resilient than we think.

You don't have to blame and shame yourself if something horrible happens to you like I innocently did. But even if you find yourself doing that, forgive yourself.

Find someone to confide in as soon as you can. You don't have to keep it a secret. You are not broken, and you don't need to be fixed. You are not what has happened to you.

Our true self (or soul) is made of love, happiness, peace and resilience and can never be destroyed. Isn't that amazing? Wisdom is always available to us. It can show up anytime to help us and guide us, as it did me when my inner voice told me to stay calm on that day.

Our feelings are always coming from our thinking and not our circumstances or other people. Having this understanding can be life-changing when we really see it.

Does any of this resonate with you?

When has your wisdom come through for you?

Do you believe that you have resilience inside of you?

Would you like to be happy no matter what?

Author Bio:

Alison Chan Lung is an intuitive, transformational coach. She has worn many hats - psychic love coach, intuitive coach and trainer, writer, speaker. However under the hats, she sees herself as someone who is curious about life, and love, and how it all fits together. She is happy to be able to share and teach what she understands about how life and love works from the inside-out.

Alison has believed we are spiritual beings having a human experience since she was young. She came from a Chinese and Irish background but grew up in Pinner near London, UK.

Her journey into personal development started with an interest in the work of Louise Hay and has been completed with her passion for the work of Sydney Banks. She has been fascinated by the workings of the soul and our connection to spirit, but is also a fan of good old common sense.

Alison founded the Soul Mate Relationship Programme in 2003 and has been fortunate enough to work with many clients who are now in loving, long lasting relationships and sometimes she gets to wear a new hat!

She has a strong desire to coach and guide clients to the best of her ability in their relationship with themselves, with a romantic partner, and with their thinking. To help them tap into their own wisdom, inner peace, resilience and happiness.

Alison lives with her partner and dog in London.

Connect with Alison:

Website: www.alisonchanlung.com

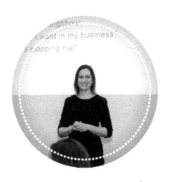

I Am A Fraud
By Elizabeth Mary Hancock

'Every time you are tempted to react in the same old way, ask if you want to be a prisoner of the past or a pioneer of the future' ~ Deepak Chopra

Have you ever felt like a fraud? Like you're living a double-life and duping those around you, including yourself?

This was me earlier this year. Life was fantastic. My business was growing successfully. My marriage was great. I had this whole work-life balance thing more-or-less figured out. I was living the dream! Then out of nowhere, old but familiar feelings began to re-surface. I started to doubt myself and question my abilities. I began to wonder why anyone would take me and my business seriously, why they'd ever want to invest large sums of money to work with me. I felt like a fraud.

I'd worked intensively on these in the past and thought I was *done* with all that crap. But when you think you've done the work, the subconscious mind always has a way of telling you otherwise.

My Story

When I was 16, I left home to live with a guy who was almost 15 years older. He charmed the socks off of me, and I fell for him big time. He treated me like a princess and made me feel important, sexy, worthwhile, confident and powerful, lavishing me with attention.

I pretty much moved in with him straight away. My parents liked him and were supportive of our relationship. Everything was perfect. Or so it seemed. However, within a month we had our first ferocious row, and he hit me. This was just the beginning of many more volatile arguments to come. In fact, if we got through a week without a row, I felt lucky and hopeful that maybe *this* time everything was going to be OK. It was a car crash of a life, but I was young, weak and became addicted to the drama and passion.

Graham never apologised for his behaviour; he never even acknowledged it, always acting as though nothing had happened. I started to lose my mind and question my sanity, believing I'd imagined every fight. I made every argument my fault, turning from happy-go-lucky into a crazy, possessive person seemingly overnight. It became my new normal; I believed living like this *was* normal.

This continued for two and a half years, escalating into greater depths of violence. There were many dinners hurled at me and the wall. He would regularly drive off in a rage of anger if he thought I'd so much as glanced at another man, often leaving me to make my own way home, and physically unleashing his wrath on my return.

Once he made me think he was going to crash the car, hurtling at top speed towards a brick wall. He slammed on the brakes just in time.

When I applied for University, he made me promise not to leave him, so I only applied for one that was local. In the end, I joined a training program at Harrods Department Store so that I could earn while learning. Graham was on a low income, and needed me to contribute to his household bills. I even spent my Nanna's inheritance on a new kitchen for *his* house.

A Desperate Cry for Help

After another terrible argument, he stormed out to the pub. I was miserable, alone, and so desperately wanted him to see how unhappy I was. It's like he couldn't even see me at all. I was trapped in my own mental hell, believing that everything was my fault. I wanted his attention, for him to acknowledge the torment I was in. So I took an overdose. When he came back, I wasn't unconscious on the floor as I'd hoped. Instead, I was trying not to be sick, and he laughed at me because I'd actually taken a load of his slimming pills – I couldn't even get that right! Many times I'd stand for hours with a carving knife in my hand, but I was too afraid to use it on myself.

Graham never hit me above the neck – it was his primary rule - so there were never any visible signs to cover up. Nobody knew what was going on, except my middle sister who, although concerned, never told a soul and didn't encourage me to leave him. Not that I would have done anyway, of course. People question why abused women stay with their partners. It's almost impossible to explain, but when you feel that you're to blame and your self-esteem is at rock bottom, you feel grateful. Grateful that someone wants you, despite all the problems you believe *you* have created. Grateful for the few times he *does* show you love because it means that you've finally done something right, finally succeeded in making him happy. And in truth, when you're buried so deep, it's hard to see a way out (or even consider the possibility that there might be).

I would have left him sooner than I did, but I felt so trapped. I finally plucked up the courage once I realised that I didn't love him anymore and I didn't want my life to be like this forever. But I was still torn. I wrote a list of reasons why I should leave, which he later found in my bag while searching for proof that I was cheating on him. He didn't believe my long working hours as an intern at Harrods were just that. You can imagine how discovering the list went down.

At one point I did leave him for two weeks while my parents went on holiday, but when they returned I moved back in with him to give him one last chance, and because I had nowhere else to go. You see, a year earlier, I'd had a massive argument with my eldest sister, and after taking her side, my parents threw me out of the house. My belongings were packed up in black plastic bags, and my childhood bedroom was re-decorated within weeks.

The Ultimate Betrayal

When I finally left the relationship for good, my parents agreed that I could move back home. However, Graham had other ideas. He would call the house at 2 am, turn up on the doorstep unannounced and plead ignorance, claiming he didn't know what he'd done wrong. And this is when my parents gave me the biggest blow of my life – the core reason why these feelings of fraud were resurfacing many years later.

They'd never asked me about the violence and abuse before; in their eyes, Graham could do no wrong. This was despite me coming home a shaking and bruised wreck the night I left him and finally told them what had been going on. When they became tired of the 2 am wake-up calls, my Mother said to me 'you have no idea what this is doing to us.'

I asked them, 'Exactly what *is* it doing to you? I'm the one who's been in an abusive relationship for the last two and a half years...' There was no love or support there for me. Can you imagine hearing that - your parents more concerned about their lack of sleep than your trauma and pain?

When I blew up about this, they said the most hurtful words they've ever uttered to me. They didn't believe that the violence had even happened; they thought I was making it up. I questioned them about the visible marks they had seen on the one occasion he'd broken the rules and left a bite mark on my chin and finger marks around my neck when he'd tried to strangle me - the night I had left. I almost wished I still had them so I could remind them of the physical proof. I can't remember what they said, but I know there were no apologies, no hugs or sympathy. I was given a very clear message that they didn't believe me.

I ended up feeling like a crazy person all over again and started questioning myself. Was it as bad as I thought? Had I exaggerated it or even imagined the whole thing? Had I brought it all on myself? Was it *really* my fault? I had always been a trouble-maker and attention seeker after all; at least that's the message I'd been given. Thoughts that I'd been resisting to rebuild myself came bubbling back up and started to cripple me again.

My life changed that day. This was honestly far worse than the abuse, the arguments, the dinners thrown at the wall, the humiliation, *everything* that had happened. This was the biggest betrayal, the most traumatic and life-changing – a few words that perhaps slipped out accidentally and without intent, but that could never be taken back – and never have been.

I lived at home for another two years. They were testing times. My parents had no idea I got into drugs and used to drink myself into oblivion. I was on anti-depressants (thank goodness) and credit them and the horse I rode as literally saving my life - he was the only one who understood, accepted and loved me, and he couldn't even talk! I slowly started to make friends again, having been forced by my ex to cut ties with my old ones. I'll always be grateful to one special friend who helped me through the dark times, and an incredible group of people who welcomed me into their fold. The fact that most of our socialising revolved around more drugs and alcohol didn't matter; I felt loved, accepted and cared for.

Eventually, I moved to London and started again - a total insomniac, still depressed, still drinking, but ready to start living my life. Very slowly I managed to come off the anti-depressants once I was in a stable relationship with the man who was to become my husband a few years later. We didn't have the smoothest journey to the altar, in fact, it was a pretty bumpy ride. I still got very drunk at times, and my self-destructive side would often raise its ugly head. It took *a lot* of work and I needed a lot of help to believe I was loveable. Learning to love me first was the most significant breakthrough on my long, tough and exhausting journey to happiness. The insomnia was debilitating and only something I've managed to crack since having my children.

Light at the End of the Tunnel

Fast forward 16 years and I'm living in beautiful Buckinghamshire with my gorgeous family. I'm happier than I ever thought possible. Yes, some days I feel frustrated and stressed, but nothing unusual for a passionate and busy entrepreneurial woman and mother.

Realising and releasing the deeply rooted fraud complex was a massive thing for me to work through and who knows if it will ever be completely gone. My programming taught me: "I am a fraud. I must be. If my Mum and Dad don't believe me over something like that, why on earth would anyone believe what I'm saying is worth listening to!'

What had kicked off the latest round of doubt and self-sabotage? An argument with my sister over the care of our parents and their situation. I realised I felt deep guilt for not being more involved in their problems, but at the same time, a part of me was still yearning for acceptance, and recognition of how they'd hurt me all those years before. Thoughts of an apology are just fantasy. I know if I ever raised this with them it would not go well. I could have spoken my truth, something I advocate for, yet I also understand that this could be detrimental to our current strong relationship. I still love my parents dearly despite all the hurt. That's part of the process. You may never forget, but who and how does *not* forgiving help? It just causes more heartache.

If it wasn't for everything I've been through, I probably wouldn't have discovered the many tools and techniques I now use as a way of clearing trauma and re-programming my mind for success. I am so grateful for my life and my experiences. I hold no hard feelings towards my ex, although I will admit to the occasional day when the lack of belief in me from my parents is something I wish I didn't have to deal with. On the flip side, it has made me the loving, compassionate and kind person I am today and has enabled me to become a pretty awesome Mum, even though I don't get it right all the time!

Whatever life throws at us, I know that with the right support we can get through it; I've witnessed it so many times. Because of my experiences, it's now my life's work to help others break through their trauma and past programming. I help them shift their beliefs and the 'Fraud Complex' or 'Imposter Syndrome', as well as many more blocks to success and abundance so that they can have the business and life they desire and deserve.

Every day I am thankful to have discovered EFT Tapping and coaching. They have been fundamental in me developing a positive mindset, taking responsibility for my feelings and actions, coming out of victim mode, undoing deep hurt and betrayal, and actualizing my dreams into reality. Little did I know that my previous corporate training role - something I thought I'd never go back to after my children - would be of use as I set up my own business and started helping others, not just myself!

With the tools I've acquired, I know I can get through anything, and with this mindset, I am making sure it happens. Maybe my Fraud Complex will *always* be there and will come back again, but I'm confident this is the last critical piece of the *current* puzzle!

Wherever your journey started or has taken you from and to, there's always *someone* willing to walk it with you. I hope for some of you, that companion is me!

Author Bio:

Elizabeth Mary Hancock aka The Wealthy Entrepreneur Coach transforms struggling and fearful but passionate coaches, consultants and practitioners into the Wealthy Entrepreneurs they deserve to be. She helps them to get more clients, charge what they're worth and feel fabulous about it! Their businesses go from average to awesome, and they achieve true emotional and financial freedom with a process that lasts a lifetime!

Liz helps her clients to dissolve their money and success blocks and go from being overwhelmed and consistently inconsistent to taking committed consistent and inspired action. Her clients go from limited to limitless so they don't just dream it, but believe it and most importantly, achieve it!

Connect with Liz:
Website: www.elizabethmaryhancock.com
Email: liz@elizabethmaryhancock.com

Hope

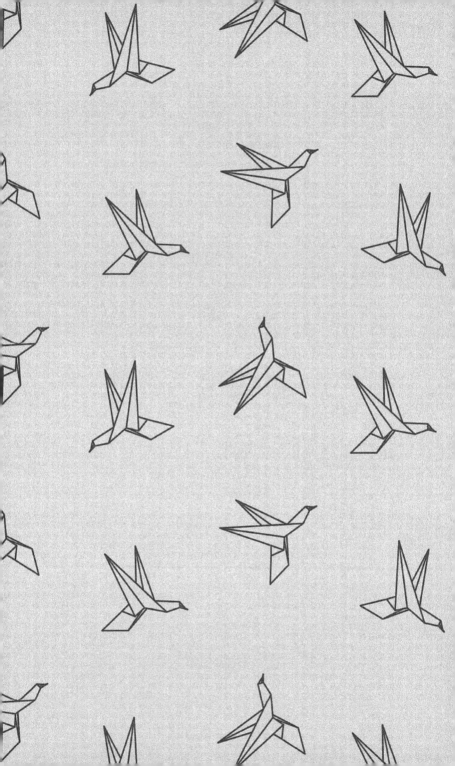

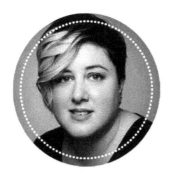

Living A Reconnected Life
By Emily Jacob

'I haven't seen Barbados, so I must get out of this'
- Tori Amos

Back in 2008, I was 34, newly divorced after ten years of marriage, and back on the dating scene. I had been out on only a handful of dates before I went out on this date. We'd spoken on the phone; I'd thought I'd checked him out. He seemed personable, and I remember being quite excited about meeting him. We went to a restaurant, we had a cocktail each to calm the nerves, and then because it was a Polish restaurant, we ordered vodka with our meal.

I remember telling him between the starter and the main

course, over a cigarette outside, that I was having a good time, but I didn't see this going further.

I didn't know that for a particular type of man, that could be a red rag to a bull.

I don't remember anything after that cigarette break. I don't remember getting home. The police later told me that according to the restaurant bill, if I had only drunk half of the vodka that was billed, I would have been several times over the legal driving limit.

At some point, I came to and he was in me. I didn't say no, and I didn't say get off. I said you're not wearing a condom. It's strange how the brain works.

I slipped in and out of consciousness. At one point I must've been fighting him because later with my psychiatrist I recalled the moment I thought I would die, face down into the mattress, his hand on my neck. That's when I froze. I remember that paralysis. Eventually, I submitted.

It was violent. He used kitchen implements. He used the attachment that the coffee grounds were kept in. I'm kinky, and he used a cane that had been left out. Nine years later, I can still see where my skin broke on my thighs from the bruising and the welts that were left.

Before he left, he made me make him a drink, and he put the ice inside me. My psychiatrist said that was a typical M.O., to reduce the bruising.

The next day, he sent me a text. He called me a young lady, said he'd had a lovely time, could we do it again.

Apparently, that was meant to confuse me and to confuse the authorities if I reported. Which I did, about a month later. It went nowhere, the CPS (Crown Prosecution Service) decided not to prosecute.

Two years later I found out their reasons.

I'd waited a month (most rapes aren't reported immediately), I'd been drinking (which should have been proof by itself of non-consent as legally I cannot consent if drunk), and he offered into evidence photographs that apparently showed me consenting (how does a picture do that? I didn't have a clear recollection of photographs being taken, although I had said in my statement I thought it might have happened).

The inability to get justice afterward had kicked me when I was already down. Two years later when I found out why, I was kicked down again.

In trying to recover, I did the things you're supposed to do. I went to victim support. I went to the Havens. I went to the

Women & Girls network. I got some one-to-one counselling, and I graduated to the group therapy programme.

I thought I was better because I'd taken my medicine. I wasn't better. I still woke every morning with the thought of him on me. I still had nightmares, and flashbacks, and often several panic attacks before leaving the house. I thought that was just my new normal, and to get used to it.

I was still numbing every emotion, through every conceivable way. Food, cigarettes, alcohol, drugs, prescription and otherwise. Cutting. I became a workaholic, working 12-14 hour days seven days a week.

I had a meltdown, a breakdown; in hindsight it was maybe a breakthrough. The medicine was prescribed again: one to one counselling, group therapy. I then also had psychiatric help for about 18 months, which incorporated many modalities including EMDR. I thought it had saved my life.

Except it hadn't. Because after, when I was discharged and told I wasn't mental anymore, I still didn't have a clue how to be in this world, this world that had betrayed me so badly.

I felt ungrateful. I'd overcome (most of) the negative coping behaviours. I'd started sleeping through the night. I didn't have panic attacks anymore. I was even weaning myself off the anti-depressants. I'd had some incredible help that had 'cured' me to the point I could say I was 'in remission', or even 'recovered'. And, yet, I didn't know how to do life, I didn't know how to be. I still didn't feel 'right', I didn't feel like I 'belonged' in the world, I still felt 'broken' and 'fragile'. I didn't trust my cure, I didn't feel connected to anyone or anything, not even myself.

I thought this was just the way life was going to be. One day at a time. Surviving. Better than before, no more panic attacks, but still, not whole, not actually living. Surviving.

I thought I was learning how to be a coach for my own business. What I found was, that in learning how to help other people, I was also learning how to help myself. I was learning how to start to feel connected to the world, to dreams, to the future, to me, again.

I learned how to stop defining myself by what had happened. I learned how to let go of the hurt, how to comfort the child in me, that defining myself as broken meant I was going to stay broken. I learned how to create a plan for a life that had tangible milestones and made me feel in control of what might otherwise have felt like an overwhelming pipe dream. I learned how to manage my internal self-talk, and reframe from negative to positive. And, most of all, I learned how to believe in myself again and find my authentic voice: not the angry hurt voice, but the voice that had been buried deep inside and saw a vision of a different world.

My mind was ready; my body was not. It seemed to want to stay in the hyper/hypo yo-yo, wanting to sleep and collapse after any minor excitement. It was becoming my Achilles heel, and I resented it more than ever, holding me back, preventing me from doing everything my head now said I could.

Then, one evening, completely unexpectedly, something clicked. I was at a women's retreat, the kind where you do lots of intensive & challenging internal personal work, not the kind where you have face masks and massages. It was an exercise in connecting with our inner vitality, our inner soul animal. I watched everyone connecting with tigers, lions, dancing, moving. And yet I was trapped, I couldn't move; I was locked, frozen, in position. The tears started rolling down my face. I realised: I hadn't forgiven my body for what had happened to me. My mind and my body were disconnected.

Up until that point, I'd been dealing with symptoms and trying to control conscious thought. And although this had undoubtedly saved my life, what I needed to do, was make peace with my body and start living as a whole human being again.

I'd found the missing piece to my recovery.

I have been working hard ever since, slowly reconnecting

my mind with my body, my body with my mind. The self-care rituals that I have put in place keep me centred, grounded and connected. It is this triumvirate of being able to self-rescue from our symptoms, re-discover who we are at our core, and re-connect to our body so we can re-connect to the world that forms the central building blocks of the ReConnected Life™ Experience that I teach.

Connection, after air, food and water, is the fundamental need for humans to express their humanity. Without connection, within ourselves, with others, with the planet, we can feel irrelevant, invisible, unworthy. Connection is as vital as the blood running through our veins. Trauma draws us into ourselves; we retreat, we cut ourselves off from others, we cut ourselves off from our true self. Learning how to reconnect, within ourselves, as well as outwardly to those close to us, and to the world as a whole, is a critical component to recovery. In fact, it has been found that the strength of our support network, our community, can determine how quickly we can recover from trauma.

I feel honoured and privileged to have discovered this pathway. The traditional narrative of trauma recovery after rape is to focus on controlling, alleviating, or removing our psychological symptoms. While the traditional routes of counselling and therapy will support us, they are often out of reach for many, either because waiting lists are so long or because we cannot afford to take a different route. However, we can create and learn the rituals for ourselves which will enable us to build our resilience and allow us to self-rescue. It's very rare also to find a recovery approach which tells us that we also need to do inner work on our thoughts, and integrate our body back into being.

Too often survivors need to fashion their own recovery path, and it can feel like an uphill struggle. I have curated the knowledge, techniques and skills so that we can be empowered to find our own unique way to our ReConnected Life™.

I call this programme the ReConnected Life™ Experience because that's what we seek, to experience a life that is reconnected. And because it's sometimes really hard to take the first step, I've created a taster experience which empowers survivors to be their own rescuer called Taste of Recovery to help them get to the place where they want to take the next steps along the pathway too.

My dream to live more than a half-life, coping one day at a time came true. It can for you too.

Reader Notes:

- Recovery from rape is far more than the treatment of our symptoms; we are whole humans and our recovery needs to reflect that

- It is possible to build resilience through developing self-care rituals
- We do not need to define ourselves as broken or fragile; we can become empowered and powerful
- When we can learn how to reconnect with our bodies we can become whole again
- And when we can authentically connect with others as our true selves, we start to connect with life and living again.
- There is a way out of this; there is a way through. There is a way to live a ReConnected Life™.

Author Bio:

I'm on a mission to support survivors in living more than a half-life, coping one day at a time, to living a full and whole ReConnected Life™. I have used my experience and the skills I developed in my recovery to create a pathway to living reconnected that goes beyond merely managing our symptoms from the trauma. I am on a mission to challenge and change the false myths that say we will be forever broken and to address trauma recovery from a whole-person holistic perspective. I'm also on a mission to end rape culture, and to speak up for survivors every opportunity I get, so you can often find me writing or speaking in the public sphere to break the silence and change the world. I'm a coach, an NLP master practitioner, an author, a blogger, a speaker, a community leader, a survivor: I'm a Badass.

Connect with Emily:

Website: www.reconnected.life
Join the free ReConnected Life Community:
www.reconnected.life/community
Connect on Twitter: www.twitter.com/ReConnectedEm
Follow ReConnected Life on Facebook:
www.facebook.com/ReConnectedLifeExperience

If you're interested in finding out more about the ReConnected Life Experience, see here:
www.reconnected.life/experience

And for free downloads and resources, see here:
www.reconnected.life/resources

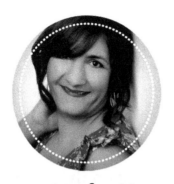

Praying for Time
By Suzie Welstead

'Hanging on to hope, when there is no hope to speak of. And the wounded skies above say it's much much too late. Well maybe we should all be praying for time'
~ George Michael

It was 25th December 2016 11.20pm. I'd had a beautiful Christmas day with my two boys and husband. Christmas had always been difficult as my birth family were no longer a part of my life. But I was so grateful to have my own family; they were more than enough.

I was heading downstairs when my eldest son stopped me in my tracks.

'I have some news you're not going to like', he said. 'George Michael is dead'.

Oh my gosh, no! I stumbled down the stairs. *Dear God, let this be a mistake.* But it was true. My idol, my legend, my hero, my saviour during tough times was gone.

Living on the Streets

Aged 17 I made myself homeless. I couldn't take the physical, mental and emotional abuse anymore. Home life was unbearable. I was isolated, controlled; I needed to break free. I desperately craved the freedom to do what I wanted, say what I wanted and be who I desperately wanted to be. I had tried - and failed –to leave many times, but this time it was for real. I'd made up my mind, and there was no going back.

The day I decided to leave was a Friday. I arrived home from school and started making the tea like always. It was my favourite - chips, beans and runny fried egg. I cooked for the family, and the urge hit me. I grabbed my white school satchel, added a toilet roll, my diary, a pen and 20p, shouted up the stairs that I was leaving then ran out of the house. Where I was going or what I was going to do, I didn't know. I just knew I had to keep running.

It must have been about 11.30pm when I started panicking. I had never been on my own in the streets at night. I could hear people coming out of the pub, and I froze. *Oh gosh, what do I do?* I was terrified. I ran to the phone box and, after scuffling through my bag for the 20p, I rang a friend or two to see if they could help me. They said no. They knew I was in a bad place and that helping me would bring shame on them and their families. I was all alone.

Luckily I had the telephone number for the Samaritans in my diary. I must have had the foresight to jot the number down when I saw it at school. I rang the number, in a state of panic and overwhelm mixed with relief and freedom. I had escaped yet fearful of where I would end up or what might happen to me. The Samaritans kept me talking and reassured me that everything would be ok. They kept me talking until a taxi collected me and took me to a refuge.

Lost and Alone

It felt strange to be in a new room, somewhere unfamiliar yet safe. I couldn't believe I'd done it, that I'd left. I hadn't planned it, but I guess I was at my tipping point. At 17 I was solely responsible for cooking, cleaning and all other household chores on top of going out to work with the added blow that I wasn't allowed to keep my wages. I knew I'd made the right decision but my mind was in overdrive -

thinking, panicking, excited, scared - I'm amazed I got to sleep.

I awoke to a loud knocking and banging on the door. It startled me; my heart jumped into my throat. I grabbed my duvet and listened at the door, relieved when I realised it was a husband looking for his wife. I sat back on the bed and, whether through shock or just the realization of what I had been through, I cried. I cried my little heart out. Tears fell and kept rolling down my face. And then I realised why I cried so hard: no one came for me.

That knock on the door made me believe that someone was coming for me, that they were looking for me, that they wanted me back. I felt that maybe, just maybe, someone cared. But they didn't. And the truth was they never did. Was I *that* bad? Was I so unlovable that no one wanted me? I was only 17 yet had never felt so worthless, unwanted and alone.

Clinging to Hope

The following morning I woke up feeling hopeful with a deep knowing that I could do this; there was no going back! A support worker came to my aid with a toothbrush and toothpaste. I will never forget how supportive and understanding she was. She asked if I wanted to ring home and made it clear that I didn't have to go back there and could stay at the refuge for 6-months. It was one of the hardest phone calls I've ever made in my life. I was nervous, sweating profusely and so glad that this was not happening face-to-face. My mum answered. I recall saying her name and thinking how little affection there was between us. She told me to come home, telling me it would all be forgotten. I told her I wasn't coming back. And that was it. She said she never wanted to see me again and slammed the phone down, affirming to me that I'd done the right thing.

The next six months passed by like a whirlwind. I felt I was living someone else's life. All I'd ever known was my parents' control and expectations, so I didn't know who I was meant to be or what I was supposed to do. Every time I went out I had to look over my shoulder for fear of bumping into someone that knew my family or me.

I wanted to understand why I wasn't loved, why I wasn't wanted, so turned to my family doctor. It turned out that me being a girl meant I was rejected the moment I was born; I already had an older sister and, with boys being highly revered in Asian culture, my parents had hoped for a son. My brother was born a few years later. This confirmed why I always felt like the odd one out in the family – unloved, unwanted and anything but special. A few days later I bumped into a family friend. She was surprised to see me. I wanted to know if my family had mentioned me, still desperately clinging to hope that *maybe* they did miss me and love me after all. Only it wasn't to be. My mum had told everyone that I had died in a car crash. My world once again came crashing down and I started to question everything, locking myself away until my 18th birthday when I was finally ready to face the world.

Praying for Time

On 8th September 1988, I turned 18 in a houseful of strangers who made me feel so special. I felt like all my birthdays and Christmases had come at once! I had never had a birthday card or present from home yet these beautiful people, in spite of hardship, had saved up and created a birthday that I would never forget. They had bought me a music centre and music that I could play, cards, food, vodka, everything they could think of to make my day special. I was immensely grateful though struggled to express this outwardly. I had no idea how to react as no one had ever done anything like this for me before. Here I was, in a room full of strangers singing happy birthday like they'd known me my whole life, something my family had failed to do. I was touched and felt honoured to have them all in my life. *Praying For Time* by George Michael came on, and I knew that in time everything would be ok.

You see, George was there again like he always had been, comforting me with his words and music. When his songs played, it was as if he was with me, the power of his lyrics and tunes easing my pain.

Now that I was 18 and an adult I had to start making important decisions about my life. It was time to move on from the refuge, leave the city and start afresh. While living in the refuge, a lady I met said she was looking for a lodger and was happy for me to move in so long as I found a job and paid my way. So that is what I did. I contacted my brother to bring me some clothes from home, he being my only link to my old life, and left the city. For a while I flitted here and there, moving from place to place as I tried to find somewhere I could establish some roots and call home. No matter where I went I never entirely belonged. I lost most of my music collection and my stereo from all the moving around. At times I felt I knew what I wanted while at other times my life felt as if I was standing still waiting for someone to give me direction.

Finding Love

Finally, I found a friend who I felt I could trust who introduced me to her mum who was so caring and kind it touched my heart. They took on lodgers but had no room for me at the time. I felt so lost and desperately unhappy where I was staying so they invited me to visit on many occasions. One day they invited me over, and while I was there one of the lodgers announced that she was moving out. Without hesitation, my friend asked if I wanted to move in. I replied with a hug and ecstatic YES. I moved in, and for the first time, I felt that I belonged, that I finally had somewhere that I could call home. I was made to feel welcome and cared for, and that meant more than words can ever describe. We had lots of fun together, lots of laughter. We looked out for each other, went partying together; life was incredible. My 21st birthday was a pivotal moment of my life. I felt happy, free and full of hope. Despite my past, I had a future that I could look forward to. And who would have thought that only six-months later I would meet the man who would become my husband and father of my children, and that we'd create the family life that I'd desperately craved as a child.

Never give up. Never lose hope, and in the words of George Michael, no matter how hard life seems, 'we should all be praying for time'.

Reader Notes:

If you are suffering any emotional, physical and/or mental abuse - *any* trauma from the past - please start writing down how you feel, little by little, step by step. Get it out of your head. Draw, write, paint - you don't have to show anybody. If you can, write every day about how you feel as your emotions can be suppressed; one day you may feel good and not so great the next. The more you write the more you will understand yourself and make the right choices for you to move forward.

I also highly recommend ringing the Samaritans. I found it very difficult to express myself early on and used Samaritans before later investing in myself to get some support.

Keep believing, have faith...and I'm always here if you need my support.

Author Bio:

Suzie is a happiness life coach with a huge passion to help create a bright and better future for her clients. She helps them explore their own happiness within them that has been suppressed by life experiences and life conditioning. Suzie herself experienced homelessness at the age of 17 to escape emotional, mental and physical abuse. She lived in a refugee for 6 months before turning her life around and embarking on a career in mental health and charity work, supporting disadvantaged teens teaching life skills and self-love, listening to the suicidal and supporting victims and survivors of domestic abuse aged 5 to 25.

Suzie now runs her own company uplifting and motivating clients to become the best version of themselves, empowering them to believe in themselves and teach them that they are enough. She believes that the next generation needs us more than ever and her mission is to help others believe to achieve, to know that they are so much more than their qualifications and that we all have gifts, life experiences and stories that we can share to help teach others.

Suzie lives in Leicestershire with her husband of 23 years and her two sons. She loves walking, water colours and spending quality time with her family and friends.

Connect with Suzie:

Instagram: suziebelieve2achieve4ever
LinkedIn: suziewelstead
Website: www.suziesunshine.co.uk

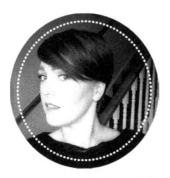

Against the Odds
By Stacy Humphris Blackley

'We all make mistakes, have struggles, and even regret things in our past. But you are not your mistakes, you are not your struggles, and you are here NOW with the power to shape your day and your future'. ~ Steve Maraboli

When I was seventeen, I made the most painful and regretful decision of my life.

I'd been with my boyfriend for over two years; he was my world. He was the one I was going to marry and start a family with; we had so many plans for our future together. Then I fell pregnant. Our baby was due after my 18th birthday on Mother's Day (of all days), and while I was overjoyed, he wasn't.

We'd spent days, weeks, months talking about names, where we would live, even down to the pushchair we would buy. Yet for him it was all a pretence; he wanted me to have an abortion. I was mortified, distraught. I couldn't understand how he could want me to do something like that or even have the audacity to ask me. He knew how badly I wanted this child.

Our families were not very supportive of our relationship. He was Hindu and me English, and despite planning both Hindu and English wedding ceremonies to appease both families, the cultural difference had created a divide. A baby certainly wouldn't be a welcome addition to either family.
I was scared and already loved this tiny baby growing inside me. I didn't know what to do so I turned to my 15-year old sister. She held my hand and said it would be okay. But she couldn't guarantee that I'd be making the right decision either way.

I finally confided in my mum. I trusted her but was still scared of how my dad would react. He wasn't approving of my relationship so would likely be unsupportive of me having my boyfriend's baby.

My dad could be violent, as I'd witnessed growing up. I knew the extent of his aggression; mum had jumped in to save me a few times. I understand now that my dad's actions and attempt to control me were his way of protecting me, to give us the best so that we didn't have to struggle like my parents did. They wanted to save me from hurt and pain, so that I wouldn't have to make decisions like the one I was facing. But being a typical teenager, I didn't listen; I didn't see the loving intent from his side. I only saw the anger when he couldn't get his point across, either defaulting to silent treatment for weeks or physically lashing out.

So I told my mum. She was devastated. She couldn't believe I had been so stupid as to get myself into this predicament. What I couldn't tell her was that this baby was no accident; it had been planned. We wanted to build a life together, or so I thought. Mum was scared for me and scared of how my dad would react, so she, from pure haste and fear, screamed at me and made me that I had no choice but to go through with the abortion. I felt alone with no parents or boyfriend to turn to, just me and the baby I wanted so badly.

A Little Girl's Dream Turned Nightmare

Since I was a little girl all I ever dreamed of was being a mum. When people asked what I wanted to be when I grew up, I always answered 'air stewardess'. It was my parents' dream for me to travel the world. But deep down all I wanted was to have someone to love, someone that would love me no matter what. Someone I could cherish and nurture. My heart ached for love. My family loved me of course, but growing up I felt that something was missing. It's like if I could love someone or loads of people my heart would burst, and the only way I could see to experience this feeling of love was to have a baby. So my dream of having a baby was coming true, yet so too was my nightmare.

I went to the doctor, and he advised a termination. At the scan I was instructed to look away from the screen, and even the sound was muted so I couldn't hear the heartbeat. Not being able to see or hear my baby, all the while knowing what I was going to put it through, was hell. I was booked in for a termination the following week and was handed a bundle of documents as I left. Me being me I had to open the file and found the scan picture. I saw my baby for the first time. She was beautiful (I always imagine she was a girl). I hugged the picture and cried all the way home in silence. I couldn't face my boyfriend; I could not talk to him.

I couldn't bear to have this baby terminated. I prayed I would miscarry so that I wouldn't have to go through with it. I felt lost and went into self-destruct mode. I stole my parents' vodka and got drunk then asked my boyfriend for hard, rough sex in the hope that it would do the job. I remember crying in pain but everything after that was a blur. I bled, I hoped it was the end, but it wasn't.

Betrayal

The day arrived. My boyfriend and I caught the bus to the clinic, but I had to get off en route to vomit as morning sickness had well and truly kicked in. We walked from there in silence; I had nothing to say to him. I was secretly hoping he would change his mind, that he would turn around and declare his love for the baby and me, that he would suggest running away together. But he did not. Instead, he waited outside while I entered the clinic, feeling more alone than ever.

In the consultation room, they told me what was going to happen before starting to sedate me. I shouted out that I was making a mistake, that I'd changed my mind and wanted to keep my baby. The next thing I knew I had woken up; it was too late. The deed had been done. I was distraught and beside myself with grief. I had killed my baby. How could I say I loved her when I'd killed her? I hated myself.

My boyfriend and I walked home in silence, and I knew from that moment that nothing connected us anymore. I didn't want anything to do with him. He couldn't understand why and wanted to work through it, but I just couldn't have a relationship with him. I knew I'd never be able to forgive him. I could never forgive myself. I arrived home and went straight to my room. For a long while life was a blur. I was severely depressed and quit college as I couldn't focus on anything. I simply felt numb.

Finding Love

Paul (now my husband) came to the rescue when I wasn't looking for a relationship. I was working in our local public house and loved it. I was starting to forge a whole new life for myself, cutting off old friendships as I couldn't face my old life. Paul was one of the regulars. I remember spilling his drink as I gave it to him and so offered to purchase him one in replacement. Weeks went by, and we got to know each other more; I really enjoyed his company. Then for a few weeks, he didn't come in. It felt strange not seeing him; our chats had become the highlight of my day. My friend asked me if there were any guys I fancied. I said, '*no but I do love Paul's company*'.

The next time Paul came into the pub, he waited for me after my shift. Unbeknown to me my friend had told him that I fancied him. He offered to walk me home. I was not keen to go home. I worked during the day and in the pub in the evenings to avoid home; it brought me back to reality and the life and memories from which I was trying to escape. So I said, 'let's go back to yours'. And we did. Funnily enough, we lived at opposite ends of the same road and never knew! We went back to his place, had a few drinks, and our friendship blossomed. It wasn't long before we were a couple.

Paul was my safe place, a place where I could be the real me. I spent hours crying on his chest while he just lay there, stroking my hair and comforting me. He was my knight in shining armour, never judging me and genuinely upset about what I'd been through.

A Rocky Road

Fast forward a few years and I discovered I had polycystic ovaries. There was slim to no chance of conceiving. I thought it was punishment for what I'd done, that I wasn't deserving of a second chance. Nevertheless, after much trying, along came our first born, Thomas. When Thomas was 15-months old, we decided to start trying for another baby, assuming it would take a long time as Thomas had.

The following month, I was pregnant. I felt blessed; a miracle had happened. But I was worried how I'd cope with two babies under the age of two. Thomas had been a challenge. He had numerous food allergies, asthma, and eczema and was later diagnosed with autism, ADHD, anxiety, and sensory processing disorder. Then when our beautiful daughter was born, we found out she had a rare heart condition. We were beside ourselves. I went into a deep depression, blaming myself, while Paul threw himself into his work.

Fast forward a few more challenging years and Paul and I married. My Dad walked me down the aisle. Despite our differences in the past, he had proven to be an incredible Grandfather and so loving and supportive of me when I became a mum. My mum and sisters helped me to get ready, and it was the most beautiful day. Our wedding felt like the first day of a new, fresh chapter of our lives. We'd been through so much, had been tested in ways that would break most couples, yet we were stronger and closer than ever.

A few years later, along came Wyatt to complete our family. What pure joy he was going to bring, another person I could love and cherish. Yet even Wyatt didn't enter the world without a fight. He was born very poorly having contracted strap b from me and almost lost his life. For a third time I was thrown into turmoil, blaming myself, thinking that again I was somehow being punished for my past mistake, that this was karma coming back to bite me. Luckily he pulled through and now brings exuberance with his zest for life.

Unconditional Love

There have been many times that I've thought what might have been with the daughter I never had. So many times I've wished I could turn the clock back. However, that experience lead me to Paul. And we have been gifted three extraordinary little beings who teach me about love, courage and strength more and more each day.

My children have been my greatest gift. They have awoken me to unconditional love and awakened the unconditional love I have for myself. Each time my mind wanders to the past they pull me back to the present, reminding me that life is happening *now*.

My journey of self-discovery means that I'm now happy with who I am and where I am going. I recognise that my power resides within me and that only I get to choose and make decisions that are right for me. My past doesn't define me, it's not who I am, and I have the power to shape each day moment to moment.

Reader Notes:

We cannot control anything outside of us, yet how we respond is our choice. We get to choose moment to moment how we show up in the world, to reclaim our power and make decisions that feel right to us.

Do the thing that scares you the most; it will lose its power over you. Many of us don't step forward because fear holds us back. We hide behind it. Yet when you do that *thing,* the fear dissolves.

Author Bio:

Stacy is a coach, badass mama and Arbonne health & wellness consultant whose gift is to not only see the potential in others but to help them unlock it. She is passionate about helping women transform from the inside out and guiding them through their deepest, darkest fears. Stacy knows that where there is pain, there is growth, and is determined to be a conscious leader to her children.

Connect with Stacy:

Facebook: www.facebook.com/stacy.humphris
Email: stacyblackley@googlemail.com

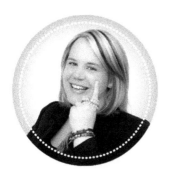

Learning to Fly
By Crystle Jones

'Just when the caterpillar thought her life was over, she became a butterfly' - Anonymous.

Have you ever looked up at the sky and wished you were free? No longer burdened or restrained, no longer this being, this person, this body, this life?

I have.

I have wanted to die a few times. I've even tried. But never have I wanted it as much as I did this summer, six weeks before writing this chapter. Never have I been so consumed by the idea of death, the kind from which you don't return.

I'm 32 years old, and my world recently imploded. My life had felt like it was on a slow decline for a long time, but this year it was as though someone took a sledgehammer to it.

Spiralling into the Depths of Despair

In June 2017 I hit rock bottom. I stormed out of my house, leaving my husband with our two girls, without saying a word. I was intent on heading straight towards the train tracks. I did not care that Russell would lose his wife and that our babies their mother; I wanted out.

On my way to the train tracks, I passed through the cemetery, and a wave of familiarity washed over me. I wanted to cry hysterically. The kind that leaves your eyes so puffy you can barely open them. I didn't care; I had made the decision that I was going to die that day. In reality, nothing mattered!

I sat on a bench bawling. My head was spinning with grief, my heart wrecked, and my soul destroyed. I wept for the woman I once was. I was so angry- how could I lose myself? What kind of idiot fucks up their life to the point that disappearing is the only answer? Who disconnects from their entire world to stop feeling anything? Who looks at their babies and wonders if there's any connection at all? Me!

At that moment there was absolutely no point in continuing; my daughters would be better off without me. How was I going to teach them to be true to who they are if I have no clue who I am? How do you connect with someone when you have spent most of your life running away from yourself?

I had let my husband and my babies down, but most of all I had let myself down. I felt guilty and ashamed of the actions I had taken. I hated everything about me. I hated my very existence. And no matter how fast or far I ran I couldn't escape the hell that was closing in on my heels.

My Dirty Secret

That morning, I'd awoken exhausted and in tears; this was nothing new. There was always a moment where I struggled to tell the difference between reality and my nightmare. In my nightmare darkness approaches, a harrowing shadow stands in the doorway. I roll over and pretend to sleep but the shadow doesn't care, it shifts closer. The walls close in and the air is suffocating; I gasp and choke. The shadow has me, and I disappear, my mind taking me to fields of peace and safety.

Finally, it's over, until the next nightmare. I feel sick and dirty, terrified and all alone.

Nothing can prepare you for the flashbacks. Nothing can prepare you for the nightmare that never ends. The nightmare that follows you around daily. I walk around with this secret, this dirty, disgusting secret. I never tell anyone about the hell I relive each day, about the nightmare, because I want my little sister to be safe, I want to be safe. He promised he would leave her alone if I played his games; they were lessons for me to learn if I ever wanted anyone to love me. This is love, the rules of love. My uncle's rules.

The flashbacks and nightmares started about eight years ago. I was eating out with a friend in a gorgeous restaurant when my world fell beneath me. The same scene from my nightmares, the same picture I see every time I close my eyes. A vast shadow, tracking the hallway to where I was sleeping or playing and finally lurking in the doorway. I feel the air closing in on me like the weight of a thousand elephants. I hold my breath because I cannot bear to smell him. I jolt and bring myself back to today. To now.

I cried for hours after that dinner date.

The next day I told Russell (my now husband) what had happened at dinner, my tone was very matter-of-fact and distant. We hadn't been dating long and I looking back he should have run. I remember him holding me, telling me I was safe. He never asked any questions about what had happened, and he never judged me; he merely allowed me to be.

I had never trusted anyone in my life, but that act of kindness made me trust him *with* my life. Not my whole life, but a considerable part of it. Something I have since learnt was just another way of relinquishing my power, my real worth. And something that I am working on daily.

Following the start of the flashbacks and nightmares, my inner child was well and truly out there. She was raging and terrified. I felt confused and scared because I knew I had been abused, I knew it happened as a child, I knew I had never told anyone, but I just couldn't remember who had abused me, until later on. Life became distorted.

I never told my parents when I was growing up and didn't tell them about the flashbacks and nightmares when these started. I never believed that they loved me or more importantly I never honestly felt loved or that they would protect me, but most of all I never trusted that they would believe me. I had a past, a history of being promiscuous (in their eyes); on several occasions, they had shamed me by calling me a slut, a whore. I believed I was a slut. I thought I was disgusting and attached my whole self-worth to sex and being with a man. I was out of control. So I never told them, I kept the secret.

Several years passed after that dreaded dinner. Life began to form. But I had become terrified of myself: what if I am an abuser? What if I am a slut? Surely I led him on, that it was my fault? I bottled up my fear and shame and continued to hide, to keep going and survive. I got married and had two beautiful girls. I honestly attempted to live life, and I honestly tried to move on. But the secret was still there, seeping into every aspect of my being. And now every aspect of my family.

Sex and Distortion

It hadn't gone unnoticed how my relationship with Russell was different to all the others I'd had. Especially the sex. It wasn't that it was easier to be intimate with him. Actually, it's the complete opposite. He once asked me 'how many people have you slept with?' I lied. I was ashamed and disgusted. If he knew the truth, he would boil his body from top to toe to rid himself of every guy I'd ever slept with and me. Or maybe I wanted to boil myself from top to toe, to peel the skin off and clean my body of the wounds I had created. Much like my self-harming scars.

I recently thought about this number, and I recall 30 (I am sure there are more). I remember the names of most of them. Some I slept with because I didn't want to be alone, others because I wanted to prove I could do what I wanted and have whomever I wanted, whenever I wanted. And some I slept with because I thought they loved me. There are four instances where the person I slept with I cared for deeply.

One of these was when I was nine or ten years old. I remember as an adult looking back and thinking, 'what the hell is wrong with you, who does that, who even knows how to do that?' I had always loved him (as much as you can when you are a child). We were playing a game of mummy and daddy (two people who should love each other unconditionally), a game I now know was also used to manipulate me when I was being sexually abused by my uncle and occasionally his son too.

This one act with my friend has haunted me most of my adult life; the confusion, the distortion, the endless questions and feelings of guilt. Did I lead him on? Did I damage him? And then there is the warped sense of what love is. This has impacted more than I could ever possibly put into words.

By the time I was in my late teens, early twenties, it was easier just to give 'it' away than to ever have to worry about 'it' being taken from me. I was disconnected, and on the odd occasion that I enjoyed it, I felt sick, ashamed and would beat myself up for days. I would talk badly to myself. I told myself that I was not worthy of love, not worthy of respect, or protection. I was damaged and broken. I believed that as a woman I wasn't supposed to feel connected or loved or respected; sex was all I was good for. I have such a warped relationship with sex and love, and the two are forever battling with each other.

I began drinking and partying at every opportunity I got, occasionally finding myself in perilous situations. One instance that haunts me is when my drink was spiked, and I woke up at a friend's house in their bed. I never had any intention of sleeping with this guy, ever! I knew he liked me, but I didn't fancy him at all, and I made it clear. But when I awoke I realised something wasn't right; my dress was half off, and my pants weren't all the way up and were inside out. I didn't know how to feel; I felt a range of emotions all at once with my mind trying to justify and make sense of it all. Maybe in my drunken stupor, I'd attempted to undress? My body didn't feel the same, it felt dirty, but I didn't remember anything and, given my past, though perhaps I'd led him on. I burst into tears and found myself consoled by this person who may or may not have raped me. I left his house feeling so confused. Surely you can trust a friend? I didn't remember anything but something wasn't right, and I felt more damaged and disconnected than ever.

The thing about trauma is your body has an incredible will to survive, and it will protect you in the only way it knows how. But being older and wiser and now having more clarity. I know in my heart of hearts I was date raped that night.

I never reported it, and until now, I had never even mentioned it.

I've taken the morning-after pill countless times, playing Russian Roulette with my health without a thought. I didn't care if I was on my period or if I even wanted to sleep with the guy, and I didn't care if I hurt my friends. I loved that I had the power. Men were easy; they were a toy to be played with. Sex became a game. And no matter what happened I could zone out, and disconnect.

Then I met Russell and he showed me I was worthy of more than just sex. When I met him, I didn't want to just sleep with him, in fact, we dated for some time before we had sex. This was very unlike me, but something was different. It wasn't easy. In fact being intimate with Russell is one of the hardest things to do, not because I don't want to, but because I do not always know how to be present and intimate with him. This is an aspect of our lives that is continually being reviewed, rewired and revisited. His kindness and accepting energy helped me to start the process of moving forward, and I began to change my perception of myself and my perception of love and sex.
He wasn't my saviour, but he did shine a light on a very dark outlook of the world.

Re-living the Past

Then two years ago my nightmare came back to haunt me again. I still hadn't told anyone (other than my husband and my friend) about the sexual abuse, or the aftermath, when my sister called to inform me that both of her babies had been abused at their nursery in South Africa. The world around me caved in, and I could feel myself fighting the urge to disconnect again. I was dizzy, like the darkness was swallowing me whole.

I tried to support my sister and her family, all while still keeping my secret. Until one day it all came bursting out. I was livid with my sister for not seeking professional help for her children, and I could see my life being relived through someone else. I couldn't let this happen. These babies needed to be protected and saved from further abuse, whether that be from others or themselves. You see that's what I was doing all this time, I was abusing myself all these years.

I stopped talking to my sister after that. I stopped having anything to do with her, because in my eyes I couldn't even begin to fathom why you wouldn't do something to help your children.

My mum stopped talking to me for six months the day I told her that my uncle had abused me; she didn't understand.

All the anger and resentment came flooding out. I was outraged at my mum for not noticing that something wasn't right with me growing up. I was angry at my sister, my dad and the world. Mostly I was furious with myself for telling them, after all, I didn't trust them. Their reaction was the exact reason I'd kept it to myself.

Then this year, the universe threw another curveball. My daughter, only 3.5 years old, disclosed that she had been touched inappropriately by her cousins, the same boys who themselves had experienced abuse. She cried so hard that night. I cried so hard that night. Russell cried so much that night. My lioness within took hold, and I made a promise that no matter what, I would not abandon her; she would be heard, believed and loved.

We called the relevant authorities and went through the motions. My daughter is so strong and most days copes well, and on days when she isn't, I am here. I am *always* here, and I will honestly do anything to help her, guide her and protect her. The case is ongoing, and we have nothing to do with my sister and her family, a further disconnect from my family but one that has been liberating. Everyone important in her life knows what has happened and how to be there for her; I will not let her live in secret or shame.

My inner child had a hard time with this attention and had to come to terms with this. These are all the things she was screaming growing up, and truthfully, for a while, she took over. My husband tried to deal with everything that was going on around him and, working in a field where disconnection is second nature; he defaulted to this coping mechanism. Disconnection was tearing us all apart, so we decided to separate.

At around this time, I started counselling because my flashbacks were more intense and I was recalling more and more. I recoiled into survival mode. The shame, disgust and sense of unworthiness overwhelmed me, and my inner child resented everyone, especially me! I began filling the void the only way I knew how by slipping into my old destructive patterns. I fell in with the 'wrong crowd', started drinking heavily, smoking, anything to numb the pain, and it wasn't long before I fell off the edge. I resorted to the only power 'game' I knew, and it was as if there were two of me. I'd somehow split myself to survive. I had to come clean with Russell with everything, and where this dark road was heading. I had to be honest with myself.

It was all too much to bear. Everything was distorted and warped, and I could no longer tell what was real and what wasn't.

A Glimmer of Hope

So here I was, losing my shit and heading for the train track to end it all.

But instead, I found the bench in the cemetery, where I was finally able to start letting go. I grieved for the secrets, the lies, the life I had lived. I raged, and after releasing so much, I began softening my gaze on myself. I had found a sense of calm and an overwhelming sense of love for my inner child who all along believed it was her fault. At that moment I promised that I would be kind to myself, that I would stop judging myself. I would learn to free my soul from the cage of abuse, and I would learn to love myself unconditionally. I decided there and then that I wanted to live my fullest life as the most authentic version of me. To follow my path and guide my family and others. I decided I wanted to live and to be the best role model for my babies. At that moment, where I had consciously chosen to die, my heart reminded me how much I wanted to live and how much I had to live for. No way would I let my uncle win, no way would I let my little girl believe that this is how it ends.

I realised at that moment that I am not a victim. I am a *survivor*!

Wow, what an insight!

The weeks that have followed my breakdown have been scary, messy and raw. I have tried not to hide who I am. This hasn't been easy because of the distortion within. I am *not* a slut, or a whore, I am ME! I am someone who spent most of my life in a world of distortion with a warped sense of reality.

I have been honest with people around me about the abuse and found an inner voice I didn't know I had. I won't lie, I have had days where I can barely get out of bed, but I still want to live. Most importantly I have been learning to love myself again, learning who I am, and learning to love myself unconditionally.

And as I sit here writing this, I know that my breakdown was really my breakthrough. Don't get me wrong, I am being real about this healing process, but my determination to know myself truly and to show my babies how to live their truth keeps me checking in. It has awakened an essence I didn't know existed within me... it has shown me my true passion and love. Really my breakthrough has saved me!

I can feel my soul and belly alight with the passion of connection, of feminine healing and love. I am a survivor but more than anything I am a warrior. My truth is now so clear and I will go on to share this with so many around me. I am alive and I intend to embrace every moment.

Author Bio:

Crystle Jones is a badass mummy, running her own massage business with huge dreams to create a well-being centre for women who have suffered trauma, where they can learn to heal and harness their divine feminine and use this energy to follow their path.

She loves learning and adding to her talents which include Angelic Reiki, Colour Therapy, Massage Therapy, Crystal Healing and soon she will qualified in Womb Massage. Her dream is to heal trauma stuck within the body or be able to offer the space for women to come and heal these traumas using methods that best suit them.

She lives in Royston, Hertfordshire with two free-spirited children and loves being creative, reading and learning, mother-nature, saving the planet one step at a time, helping others and teaching her babies to live their truth. She is best described as being airy fairy; and yes she does believe in fairies and angels.

Connect with Crystle:

Email: info@balance-me.co.uk
Web: www.balance-me.co.uk

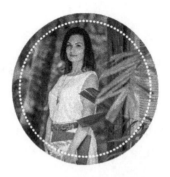

Navigating the Wilderness
By Antonina Andreeva

'Heavy is the crown and yet she wears it as if it were a feather. There is strength in her heart, determination in her eyes and the will to survive resides within her soul. She is you. A warrior, a champion, a fighter, a queen.' - r.h.Sin

'Where the hell am I?!' were my first thoughts as I opened my eyes. The ceiling looked nothing like the one at the flat. I felt dizzy and woozy, probably due to the amount of alcohol I drank the previous night at my friend's party.

A sense of dread descended upon me, planting itself firmly in my tummy. I rubbed my eyes and looked around to familiarise myself with my surroundings. It appeared that I was in a bedroom, tucked in bed, in a house that wasn't mine. 'Ok, a good start I suppose,' I thought to myself trying to calm the feeling of arising panic alerting me that something was wrong. Very, very wrong.

I looked around once more and started to realise that this room was vaguely familiar.

'Oh this is my ex-boyfriend's place,' I thought to myself,

Ex-boyfriend being a somewhat glorified description of our relationship. We were neither on nor off, rather somewhere in the middle.

Undefined.

Un-labelled.

Unspoken.

Unsaid.

I scrunched my nose and willed the recollection of yesterday's events. Last I remembered, I arrived at a mutual friend's party - a brutish from my birth country. If I was completely honest with myself, it wasn't something I wanted to do, but in my head, this was better than staying home alone. Plus, I secretly wished that I would have a chance to speak to A, the un-defined ex.

He was a boy with peculiar morals that were strong and weak at the same time, creating an air of mystery that enticed me to him no end. I thought I could be the one who could change him, get him to see the error of his ways and that he'd fall in love with me.

A few weeks prior we had had a massive falling out whereby I said some hurtful things in the heat of the moment, after which he vowed to get revenge. I never intended for us to fall out, and recognised my part in the argument. We hadn't spoken since and in my mind going to the party would be the perfect opportunity to make amends. I felt guilty for saying the things that I'd said but wasn't confident enough in him answering my calls or writing to him to apologise.

All of this was swirling in my head as I headed out, filled with anxious butterflies and further anxiety as none of my friends were going to be there. The nerves were getting the better of me.

Battling the Unknown

Once I'd arrived it quickly dawned on me that I'd made a mistake. It was 90% boys with only one other girl (I was too naive to recognise that she was a hired exotic dancer). The boys were displaying their usual bravado. Drinking, cracking sexist jokes and pretending to be grown men. It was unsettling. And yet, I stayed. My confidence had already been destroyed by my previous relationship, and I needed a man to prove my worth, so my inner voice had convinced me.

A friend of A's offered me a drink. I accepted, hoping it would calm my nerves. I remembered him looking at me and smiling and then nothing......

And now, I am in this room.

Irrational panic rose again. 'How much did I drink last night?!' I thought to myself. Suddenly, someone burst into the room. It was the boy who handed me the drink. He brought me some liquid and a sandwich. I asked him what he was doing here and what happened at the party. 'Oh, you drank too much and passed out. We had to carry you here' he answered, a little too swiftly, looking away.

Ashamed of the fact I got myself into this mess, I started getting dressed when it dawned on me....I was naked.

What *has* happened?!

What have I done?

Who was I with?

I came out of the room to see if I could gauge the ex's reaction. I couldn't. My head was spinning, and he was unreadable as always. Plus, with all his friends crashing at his place, it was hard to see past the usual adolescent bravado.

I had no choice but to flee in shame.

How can I have gotten myself into this situation?

How could I have possibly drank myself into such a stupor that I don't remember the last 8-10 hours of my life? Between entering the restaurant and waking up in the flat, I drew a complete and utter blank on the events of the night.

I was utterly disgusted with myself.

The dreaded feeling in my stomach was growing bigger by the minute and by the time I reached my house it had turned into a full-blown anxiety attack.

'I can't possibly share this with anyone,' I thought to myself. 'No one will believe me'.

This was the kind of situation your parents warned you about, that you'd read about in teen magazines and bright in-your-face typography in student leaflets.

And yet, here I was, in the middle of a nightmare.

In a bid to stop the panic that encroached me, I scraped together some pennies and headed to the nearest corner shop for cigarettes. I had coursework to hand in by Monday, so decided to complete it to distract me from my thoughts.

Trouble is my computer refused to work, my cards kept getting declined, my hands were shaking, and all I wanted to do was throw up the events of the night before.

Throw up until I expelled every last drop of that night and my decision to go along and see A. Throw up my weakness, throw up my helplessness. Throw up my guts and disgust.

In the coming weeks, I began to have intense flashbacks. I would wake up hearing someone say my name and breathe heavily into my ear. Bolting up in the middle of the night covered in cold sweat, I started to question my sanity.

I stopped going to college and instead barely left the house, self-medicating to go to sleep which further fuelled my paranoia. Unable and too ashamed to share my secret with anyone, I was slowly driving myself crazy. Every time I went to bed, my room would start spinning, and I would get heart palpitations which made me feel like I was going to die.

At this point, it would have been a *much* more comfortable option, for I wasn't really living, instead a prisoner of my mind and an experience of which I had no recollection.

My only solace at the time were spiritual books, especially *Conversations With God.* The main character spoke of the fact he could hear God. I was convinced I could hear The

Devil. Panting heavily in my ear each night, asking me if I was asleep and then laughing maniacally. I might as well have been possessed. Occasionally, I would become aware of another voice. It had a different quality to The Devil. It spoke with encouragement and asked me to keep going. It sounded and felt full of love. I was convinced this was the voice of God. This is the voice that kept me going.

Uncomfortably Numb

I remember one day a friend coming over and saying to me: 'You are a shadow of your former self. Go home, get better'.

And yet, when I reached out to my parents they came back with 'you have a month rent left on your contract, couldn't you complete on that and then come?' I felt utterly abandoned by those I loved. It was as if I could trust no one, not even myself.

Finally, after pleading with my family, I went home. In their fear of what might have happened (they'd reached out to my friend to get some info), their reception was icy. Their hostility affirmed what I already believed to be true, that I was indeed hopeless, useless, it was all my fault.

I began to see a doctor. First, a hypnotherapist who wanted to regress me, then a psychiatrist who prescribed a whole range of pills, from antipsychotic to the most potent anti-depressants & sleeping pills on the market. I put on weight, left my course at Uni and became idle. I remember looking up at the Spring sky one day and thinking 'oh, sun, how nice'. In my desire to run away from my pain, I had rendered myself completely numb. I now had NO feelings at all.

That moment I made a decision. I decided that I couldn't go on like this any longer. Fat, guilt-ridden and broken. Ashamed of being myself, of my body and my life.

Escaping to India

By chance or perhaps by Divine Synchronicity I had the opportunity to head to India. I decided to take it. It was the perfect escape from my life, a chance to disappear. I remember weighing up my options. My knowledge of India was somewhat narrow and limited, yet my life was even more narrow and limited. It was a no-brainer.

Once in India, I got the culture shock of my life. We were in the Southern part of the country, headed to an Ayurvedic Farm. I decided to use this opportunity to get off the meds once and for all. They kept me drowsy, blocked up and idle.

There, I started yoga, eating vegan and journalling every night. It took a little over a week to no longer rely on exhaustion to get me to sleep or pray to the Gods of anxiety that I wouldn't get another panic attack. I started smiling and almost enjoying life.

Then, I was given the opportunity to visit Amma, a living, hugging Saint. The Divine Mother. It would be my first time venturing outside my comfort zone and away from the patrol of my family. I was told she would whisper something into my ear, something that was meant only for me.

I was excited. For the first time in more than a year, I had something to look forward to. *I was excited*! Wow!

Eagerly I set out on a trip across the state of Kerala to meet Her. We took cars and more cars, and buses until we arrived at her proverbial doorstep. She had built an Ashram, a temple of sorts, while travelling and blessing all over the world. This was one of the times she was going to be spending time in her hometown. A cause for celebration in the locality.

Seeing the Light

The minute I stepped onto the territory of the Ashram, I experienced a feeling of familiarity. I searched my mind to find confirmation. It then occurred to me that the answer I was seeking wasn't to be found in my memory but my heart. It had been a while since I'd listened to or connected to it; the pain was too much. Here I was being asked to drop into my heart and....*hope*.

I didn't know at the time that the Divine Mother was already working with me.

I complied.

And moved a little further along the endless queue of pilgrims.

While waiting, I realised that when I believed, I could hope.

Hope that despite and in spite of what happened there was something grander than my comprehension at work. I allowed this feeling to settle into my heart and the line moved again.

My heart went ping as if to say: 'Hey if you can Believe and you can Hope, you can Trust. Maybe?'

'Mmmm Trust. That's a biggie,' went my internal dialogue.

I thought to myself, what's the *worst* that can happen? After everything I'd been through I realised I couldn't *not* try Trust on for size.

As soon as I made this very declaration my turn came. I was thrust up to the altar and in front of her. The Black Madonna herself. She was beautiful and chubby, safe and powerful all at the same time. It was almost a cognitive dissonance. To the outside world, she looked like a momma. Someone on whose breast you wanted to rest. Someone on whose shoulder you wanted to cry. Her energy was palpable.

She pulled me close for a hug. Time stopped. Amma whispered a phrase in my ear and let go. It sounded gibberish to me. After composing myself, I walked off the stage.

The truth was, I was still the same, and yet somehow I was different. In the moment of our hug, it *finally* dawned on me; I was okay with not being okay. I would no longer try to fight it, medicate it, work on it or hypnotise the shit out of myself to not be with it. I was even okay with not fully knowing what happened to me that night and equally, being accepting of what had.

Finally embracing not being okay and allowing myself to feel the discomfort as it arose was a significant step to wholeness.

It still took me another ten years to find my version of Whole. However, that moment with Amma was the beginning of a new and more liberating chapter of my life.

Reader Notes:

Acceptance is a huge part of moving through trauma. Until you accept that you are not okay, that you are not where you want to be, you will not be able to get to the other side.

When you are healing, it is essential to give yourself time and space to process everything that comes up. To the outside world, it may look like you are stalling, going backwards or not making progress. However, this is about you and your experience.

Seek a trusted friend, coach or health professional to be your guardian and your boundary keeper if you cannot master it for yourself at that moment.

Know that no matter how dire the situation might seem at the time, there is always light at the end of the tunnel. Sometimes the Soul may choose to experience pain as a way of elevating consciousness.

Ask yourself:

What support do I need in:
  1) Body
  2) Mind
  3) Soul

What does this support look like for me?

Where can I receive it from?

What am I resisting?

Author Bio:

Antonina is a Soul DNA Coach and Mentor for Awakened Purpose Driven Women. She works with Spiritually-minded people, empowering them to create the necessary changes to build a life that looks good from the outside and feels good on the inside.

Antonina passionately believes the world would be a better place if more people were truthful and honest about what sets their heart alight.

Her big mission is to assist as many women as possible to be truly happy and at peace with themselves. To become fully realised in their life and their work. To come together to heal, grow and step into their most potent, powerful self.

This will create a shift on a humanity level, redistributing the wealth into the hands of those who need it heralding the start of a New Earth.

When she is not coaching clients, she's likely found travelling to faraway places, in communion with the elements at the nearest beach, or wrestling her six-year-old into bed.

Connect with Antonina:

FB: www..facebook.com/TheCoachinista
Instagram: www.instagram.com/thecoachinista
Twitter: www.twitter.com/thecoachinista

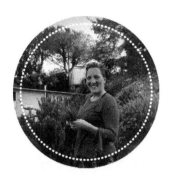

Addicted to Love
By Tara Mestre

'No matter how difficult and painful it may be,
nothing sounds as good to the soul as the truth.'
- Martha Beck

I'm sitting here trying to write a chapter on abuse and struggling. Do I want to re-live history? Resurrect ghosts from the past? It seems like such a distant memory that a part of me refuses to go there; I don't want to revive the horror that enslaved me in a living nightmare for so long.

The nightmare that never seemed to end and ate away at my soul. Every. Single. Day. A nightmare that dominated my waking life and invaded my dreams; there was no escaping it.

And then I realise I have to write this chapter because it is proof that even when you think the nightmare is never going to end, it does.

My First Love

I spent most of my late teens and twenties consumed by my ex-boyfriend. Having met him initially at 14, we became an item at 17 and stayed together for what must have been 5 or 6 years. I don't remember. I just remember he was my first love and I fell hard.

We were kids really, but that didn't diminish what we had. We found each other, and that was all that mattered. Our relationship was all-consuming, and the early days were spent showering each other with love and affection, hanging out and doing all of the things you do when you think you have finally found that person that completes you.

I was flattered by his attention, honoured even. Having spent most of my teenage years looking for a boyfriend, I had finally found The One, and I wasn't about to let anything get in my way.

I had incredible parents who always encouraged me and told me I was capable of anything. They praised me and affirmed that I was destined for great things. He, on the other hand, was born to a young mother with an abusive husband and grew up feeling like he was a mistake and a nuisance.

His home life was very different to mine. Not necessarily unhappy but different. He had a very large family, including his extended family, where everyone was involved in each other's business, and importance was put on material things. I came from a family of four with no extended family and had a very different outlook on monetary value. The differences were immense yet, in the beginning, love conquered all.

When Love Becomes Bitter Sweet

Very soon I began to see a jealous side. An aggressive side. A possessive side.

'No you can't wear that.'

'I don't want you going out without me.'

It started small but eventually got more sinister to the point that if I even looked at another guy, I was accused of being a slut, a whore, a cheat.

I remember the first time he hit me. We had been out with friends, and I had commented about a muscly bouncer. I hadn't said I was attracted to him, merely commented on his physique to a female friend. He overheard me. He left.

I found him at my house at three in the morning banging the door to be let in. He proceeded to follow me to my room and then grabbed my hands and kicked me so hard that I lost my breath for a second. I was shocked. I was scared, and as he sat in my kitchen with a knife in his hands, I feared for my life. I did the only thing that I could. I rang his father, and he came.

We broke up. But not for long. I loved him. He was my best friend. The man to whom I lost my virginity. My 'soulmate'. He was damaged and hurting, and I was going to be the one to fix him.

Little did I know at the time that this wasn't possible. You cannot fix anyone.

We stayed together for three more years, breaking up more times than I can count. I left the country to go to University in England and then one day I realised I'd had enough.

I couldn't put up with the jealousy, the control, the comments about my appearance. I understand now that those words about my weight led me to despise my body for more than a decade.

I realised that if I had any chance of being who I wanted to be, and living the life that I desired to live, I had to leave him. Our whole lives were already planned out. We were going to move to Australia far from his family and live on the beach.

Alone.
Together.

But my eyes had been opened by my university experience, and I knew deep down that I had to be with someone who loved me and who wouldn't verbally and physically abuse me. So we parted ways. I was heartbroken.

He was too, and also extremely angry.

A Fresh Start

Life went on, and I planned a trip to South-East Asia with my friends. A new beginning. A fresh perspective. Maybe some fun.

The summer was amazing. We travelled and explored, and my passion for travelling was born.

And then one day I saw him.

As I walked across a crowded bar on a beautiful tropical island in Thailand, he was there.

He saw me.

And my heart stopped. *Surely this wasn't real. How could he be here!*

We greeted each other like lovers, amazed that we had found each other. I was in a state of shock, happy yet wary. What followed was two days of bliss. We came back together and fell in love again.

Until the third night.

The Return of Past Demons

I went out with my friends, my beautiful independent girlfriends who had always stood by me and told me I was better than this.

We had drinks. We danced. And he arrived. Drunk. Angry. And the words started.

Menacing. Whispering in my ear.

'You're a slut. You're a whore.'

The music was loud so no one else could hear but my face said it all, so my friends and I left.

Back at the hotel, I cried and realised nothing had changed. He was still the same person. I showered trying to wash those words away.

There was a knock at the door. It was him.

He begged me to come upstairs so he could apologise. I believed him. I walked up wearing nothing but my towel. We walked into his room, and he locked the door.

Immediately he pushed me to the ground, grabbed my arms and told me how ugly and fat I was. How nobody would ever want me. How pathetic I was.

I braced myself because I knew I was going to die and he was going to kill me. I knew he was going to rape me. I knew this was how it was going to end.

Yet somehow, by some miracle, I broke free. And I ran, hurriedly unbolting the door, screaming as I ran past his friend in the corridor. I went back to my room, laid on my bed, and cried.

Looking back now, I was in shock. I got up the next day, and we left immediately, the bruises on my wrist serving as a reminder of his hatred towards me.

It took me a very long time to get over this. Unbelievably I went back for more, more times than I care to admit. I loved him, and despite what he did I needed him. His words had left a scar on my soul, and I believed them to be true. I felt grateful that he wanted to be with me when no one else would.

Walking Away

We stayed in this dysfunctional relationship for a while longer until one day I met my beautiful partner Ben. I discovered what it means to be with someone who only wants the best for you. Someone who loves you just the way you are. Someone who would never raise a hand to you.

When I think back to this time, I realise it made me who I am today. I am a strong independent woman. I love my body. I know I am amazing and I have no problem saying that.

The man I fell in love with did not feel that way about himself. He thought of himself as nothing, he believed he was nothing, and his anger was towards himself, not me. Now I understand and can think of him with compassion and love.

He was broken. Perhaps he still is, but just because someone is damaged, it doesn't mean it's your job to fix them. Neither is it OK to tolerate their abuse.

For anyone reading this who thinks *yes, but once I fix him it will all be OK*, remember my story. If a man diminishes and belittles you, calls you names and abuses you in any way, listen to the warning signs, see the reality of the situation, and walk away. Keep your head high and walk away.

And that's my story. Yes, it was a hard time. But it's in the past, and as I look at my beautiful son and gorgeous partner, I know that it was OK to have experienced this. From the darkness came light. My journey was always going to lead to this, and I know that the past cannot hurt or define me in any way. Rise, strong sister, for it is us that hold the light for those who are in darkness right now.

Reader Notes:

You're past is your past. It does not shape your future in anyway. Take a deep breath and say out loud 'Every day is a change for a new beginning. I let go of my past and honour who I am today'.

Physical abuse can have lasting implications. Speak to someone and allow your body to let go of this hurt. Do not carry it around with you and allow it to define you.

Look how far you have come. Too often we look at how far we have to go. You are here now. That is enough.

Author Bio:

Having swapped city life for rural living in northern Spain, Tara is first time mama, a seasoned yoga aficionado, and is passionate about yoga, women's wellness, and holistic living. She is a firm believer in self-care, incorporating yoga and essential oils into her daily routine.

Connect with Tara:

Website: www.taramestre.com
Instagram: @yogimamalove
Or join her women's group on FB: @yogimamalove.

Love

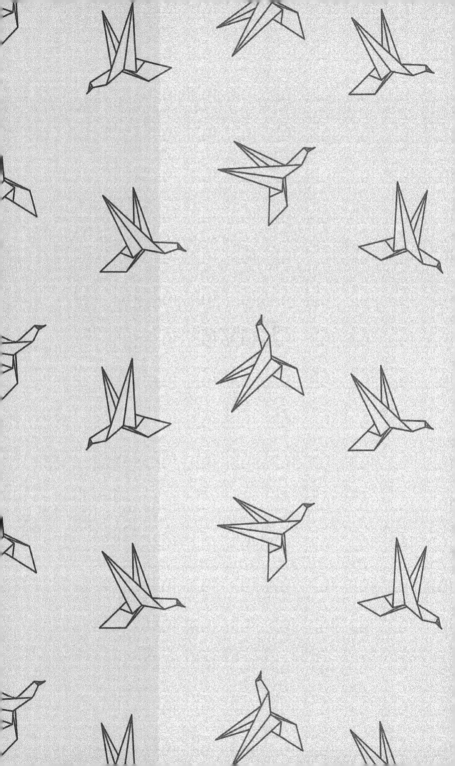

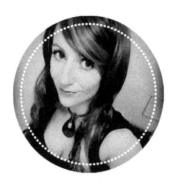

The Child Within
By Stacey Ann Coyne

'Spread love everywhere you go. Let no one ever come to you without leaving happier.' - Mother Teresa

By the divine powers of the Universe you have been drawn to this book, to my story, right here, right now and that is no coincidence.

My name is Stacey Ann Coyne. I am a self-taught survivor who has risen above more than 15 years of addiction, high levels of mental, physical and sexual abuse, PTSD, depression, anxiety and many medical diagnoses. I have taken all of my past experiences, searching deeply to discover the meaning and strength in each one.

I know first-hand a person's belief and mindset can make it possible to overcome even the most unthinkable trauma. At the age of 28, I surrendered to the beat of the universe. This ignited a fire inside my soul allowing me to pass the flame along to others and set the world ablaze with light and love. However, my life was not always so full of positive inspiration.

This is a glimpse into my journey of self-love. In sharing this, I hope to awaken your soul that, regardless of where you are in life or where you have been, you can CHOOSE to break free from limiting beliefs, rise above and tap into your inner child and become fearless in your pursuit of life!

Self-Love

Are you able to lay your mind and body bare, unprotected within its truth?

Or do you cringe at the feeling of being exposed?

Are you able to look in the mirror and see beyond the flesh transporting YOU?

Or do you attack yourself with critical thoughts becoming your own worst enemy?

Are you able to sit alone in the empty moments and enjoy the company you keep?

Or do you clutter your time with senseless distractions?

How can we truly love others if we don't first love ourselves?

What is essential for true love cannot be seen by the human eye. Love must be felt from within your own heart before passing it on to another. Don't be blinded by your eyes or fooled by your ears.

All your answers sit far beyond the skin. All your answers are within.

Who Are We?

Take a moment to close your eyes and envision the pure, innocent child you once were. The child who lived before the arms of an egotistical world wrapped themselves around you, obstructing your true vision.

Do you remember her? A magnificent pure soul that lived before being labelled, judged, and tainted by a seemingly unforgiving world. The child who saw life in all of its exquisite beauty and had no fears.

Perhaps you feel sorrow in your heart as you begin to recall the child you once were and still are. Go beyond the sorrow. Dig deeper than the pain, and I promise you can awaken her. A child filled with love, hope and endless opportunity. This child is the essence of who you are.

For me remembering my inner child was extremely difficult, until recently. I knew she still lived somewhere within me, viewing the world in all its beauty, enjoying every moment to its fullest. Yet, with every passing year, it was easier to lose sight of her, to let her slip into darkness. My soul became heavier and heavier, paralysed by the weight of so many labels, opinions, self-doubt, anger, sadness, rape, addiction, and pain until one day I awoke, and had no recollection of that once pure and loving little girl I was.

She had become a fading memory that was almost gone. Lost from a childhood that seemed never to have existed. Memories of a little girl trying to understand abuse, trying to understand love, trying to understand life. All this confusion left sadness and fear lingering for what seemed like forever.

Searching to remember the beautiful innocent child I once began a lengthy process of mixed emotions erupting in layers from years of confusion.

The first memories to arise were of a tiny girl curled up in a ball and hiding in a corner, wedged tightly between the wall and a radiator. Her hands pressed firmly to her ears as she would sing in her mind to block out the bangs and sounds of anger that echoed from her father's rage.

Was this the child I was searching for?

Next was an overweight 10-year-old standing alone on the playground. Red frizzy, untamed hair that matched perfectly to her pale freckled skin and glowed in the sun's reflection. Fatty! Ugly! Freak! Vibrations of sounds echoed from venomous words causing tears to pool within her mind, tears she withheld from pouring out of her beautiful blue eyes. Questions of her physical beauty lingered on.

Was this the child I was searching for?

A 13 year old little girl who should have been at home playing with dolls, yet here she was, lying naked in a bed, scared and ashamed, feeling exposed and terrified of what was about to happen. Tears ran down her cheek as a man took a piece of her soul she was not willing to give.

Was this the child I was searching for?

I can recall this little girl's sorrow vividly, deep in the depths of my heart; because she is me. A little girl not prepared to repel the world's harsh ways, judgment and ridicule. Instead, absorbing it all like a dry sponge dipped into water. Soaking up every ounce of abuse, every laugh, and every label I was given.

Unknowingly blind to the strength and power I held within, it became effortless to allow the cruel world around me to take residency within my mind and soul.

At a tender young age feelings of anger and confusion poured through my veins every day. Feelings piled up, one on top of another, creating so much pressure that a slight glimpse in the mirror set off a frenzy of self-sabotage from my subconscious. Freak, ugly, stupid words spiralled around my head day after day.

These words turned into my perception, creating feelings that hurt beyond measure. Feelings that embedded themselves into my core and solidified from that point on how I viewed my reflection.

Negative emotions so intense that I would have done anything to numb the pain. A floodgate of confusion and self-doubt created an endless void within my soul, one that I desperately began cramming false ideas of love into for decades. Paving a long road of addiction, abuse, eating disorders, and self-sabotage that laid the path for a long destructive journey.

Surely these memories weren't of the child I was searching for?

Where was she and how would I ever find her with no recollection of her pure love?

A lost child

For as long as I can remember, my soul felt like an aching, empty, bottomless pit. Like a hungry heart begging to be fed. A feeling that I was sure some outside source would fill and make me complete.

At a young age, I began gorging all of my insecurities with anything that would take my mind away from myself, latching on for dear life to every destructive angle I could grasp.

At age ten food numbed my pain. Rushing home from school I'd spend countless days sitting in front of the TV eating my thoughts away.

At 11 bulimia brought me comfort, giving me complete control over my eating issues, or so at least I thought.

At 12 drugs and alcohol obstructed my view, the absolute perfect potion to numb the pain burning into my every thought.

At 13 crystal meth opened up a whole new dimension, the ultimate path of no return that forever altered my life.

At 15 destructive relationships began taking over my every breath, creating strong ideas of false love and happiness.
At 16 a well-calculated man of highly decorated authority entered my life, beginning a long 5-year experience of unthinkable mental, physical and sexual abuse.

By the age of 18, the little girl I so desperately wanted to recall was lost. To hide her innocence from the cruel world of destruction I pushed her so far away, forgetting she even existed. I took all of my feelings and encapsulated them in a hard shell that wouldn't allow anyone's thoughts or opinions to penetrate.

I stood strong and unbreakable because I no longer cared about anything. I had become my own worst enemy and survival was my only concern, bouncing from one destructive behaviour to the next and setting the tone for a long adventure into a deep, dark and seemingly hopeless life.

A Crystal Palace

Dreams that were never dreamed. Endless nights that blurred into days, weeks, months and even years. All my feelings trapped in an infinite circle of confusion, pain and sadness. Year after year experiencing one horrific, unthinkable event after the next. It seemed as though no matter which way I turned, I couldn't escape. Did I even want to?

I often sat for hours on end daydreaming of what life could have been like, countless notebooks filled with internal cries for help. All were portraying a little girl who was seemingly lost along with her path, suffocating in a cloud of smoke by the opinions of others. A core so broken that hate and blame were the easiest ways to get through the day.

How did I let my life slip away into a world of darkness?

How did I become so numb to everything around me?

How did I let a man rape my mind and body for so many years before I spoke up?

How did I let others determine my worth with their words?

How did I hate myself so much?

When did addiction become more beautiful than life?

When you don't know any other way, where do you start?

The only thing that kept me alive was a glimmer of hope. A small memory of a once happy little girl that I could barely locate. A little girl who always smiled, who loved music, nature and making people laugh. Yet I couldn't feel her inside, no matter how hard I tried.

Downward Spiral

At 28 years old I was drowning in a pool of confusion barely able to breathe. On Dec 04 2009 my world took its hardest hit. That night, in a small back closet, my father tied a rope around his neck and took his life, a decision that would forever alter mine. Yes, I endured a horrific childhood at his expense although he was still my best friend and biggest hope of finding that beautiful little girl I once was. But he was gone, and so was the faith of ever unearthing her. His death gave me the perfect victim role, the perfect excuse to wallow in my own demise, the perfect reason to let myself die.

What I didn't know was that the universe had a much grander plan for me than my own.

Death for Life

One early morning, six months after my father's death, I walked past my bedroom mirror and caught a glimpse of a stranger staring back at me. Stopping dead in my tracks, I locked eyes with this unrecognisable reflection.

Who was I and what had I become? A drug dealer addicted to meth for what appeared to be my entire life. A tarnished soul that was almost drained empty, covered by a deteriorating body.

Is this really what I was meant to be? Why did I always choose self-sabotage?

What was love? What was life? Who was I? Why was I still alive?

Questions that had poured through my mind numerous times before were furiously screaming in my mind with more purpose and love than I had ever felt.

Staring deeply at my reflection, searching for that glimmer of hope, a single tear glistened as it pooled in the corner of my eye and gently released down my cheek. I hadn't cried for many years, not even at my father's death. It was within that moment I felt a calling deep within my soul telling me there was something more for me in this life, but I had no idea the magnitude of what it was.

At 28 years old the only life I knew was about to change forever.

A Power Greater than Me

Later that day an immense pain surged through my stomach, a pain I had never felt before. I ran to the bathroom and dropped to my knees, my face engulfed with a deep burning sensation and my throat tight and narrow leaving me gasping for air. After about 10 minutes the feeling slowly subsided and left me so weak I could barely pull myself off the floor. Grasping onto the sink, splashing cold water on my face and locking eyes once again with my reflection, a single thought flooded my mind: 'you're pregnant.' Staring into my own eyes for what seemed like hours, this one thought pounded every cell of my body. The certainty that I knew terrified me more than anything I had ever done.

It was that morning that a divine power came over me, and in my lowest of low points my soul awakened from an eternity of sleep. Was this the universe's answer to my prayers for death?

I sat alone that day at the doctors, my heart pounding and my mind racing with a million thoughts on what to do if this was real. I can remember the feeling when the doctor confirmed I was three months pregnant. At that moment I faced the hardest choice I would ever face:

The choice of life or death.

I was in no place to bring a life into this world, but I was also in no position to take one either. It was then that I surrendered to the Universe and asked for guidance from a power beyond me.

An Angel is Born

On Jan 19th the most beautiful soul entered this world. From a divine gift far more significant than me I gave birth to a healthy beautiful baby girl. When my father arrived in heaven, he chose the purest, sweetest angel he could find and sent her to me. Her love was the only vibration strong enough to break through my barriers, to teach me how to love myself and others.

My long journey of self-destruction lead me to the most beautiful self-discovery. Learning to forgive even unthinkable actions, to let go of anger and egoistic thoughts, allowing a new world of abundant beauty and love to be perceived.

My daughter was sent to this earth to awaken my inner child and in the process bring joy, laughter, healing, understanding and an abundance of unconditional love to everyone within her path.

The Secret

Often in life, we are programmed to count our sorrows rather than our blessings. The secret to creating a better life is feeling deep gratitude for all you have, not just what you want. I am no different than you or anyone else. The only thing that sets people apart is what we choose to focus on. What we choose for habits and what we choose to believe. You can be a victim or a warrior; the choice is yours.

Today I view life as a never-ending journey that is continuously evolving and bringing forth new habits and knowledge. I now wake up every single day to inspire people to find their inner child. To teach others how to discover self-love, how to become visionaries, and how to live life to their fullest potential regardless of their past. Spending my most recent years studying the unseen laws of the universe, nutrition and fitness has lead me to create Mind Body Image ~ Fuel your Life, a company bringing positive mental, physical and nutritional fuel to the lives of others.

I invite you to join us in creating a community filled with fearless women lifting one another to rise and take control of your destiny!

Author Bio:

Stacey Ann Coyne is an uplifting * Badass * visionary who, after overcoming 15 years of drug addiction, abuse, PTSD, depression, anxiety, countless medical diagnoses, rape and sexual assault, surrendered to the beat of the universe to ignite the fire inside others and set the world ablaze with light and love. Her driving force and most valuable 'title' is being a mother to her six-year-old daughter.

She is a true inspiration, a self-taught survivor using the Laws of the Universe, Inner Guidance, Spiritual Growth, Energy, Meditation, NLP, Nutrition and Fitness as her tools to recreate not only her life but the lives of others, filling them with everlasting love, health and meaning. She believes a person's mind and thoughts are the most valuable tools to overcome even unthinkable trauma. Stacey's passions have guided her to build Mind Body Image, a company bringing positive mental, physical and nutritional fuel to the lives of others.

Stacey is a Health & Wellness Specialist, Author & Motivational Speaker, Child Advocate for Real Food. Founder and CEO of Mind-Body Image, Chiropractic Assistant, Stott Pilates Instructor, Reiki Practitioner and NLP Practitioner.

Her most recent speaking engagements include Boston State House ~ overcoming adversity, Quarterly UPS Woman's Business Leadership Groups ~ Health and Wellness, Walpole Library, Mind Body Image ~ Fuel your Kids, and March against Monsanto ~ GMO rights advocate.

Connect with Stacey:

Website: www.mindbodyimage.org
Facebook: www.facebook.com/MindBodyImage

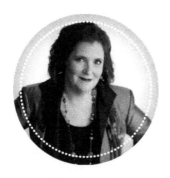

From Committed Underachiever to Fearless Entrepreneur
By Alison BW Pena

'Make the most of yourself by fanning the tiny, inner sparks of possibility into flames of achievement.' - Golda Meir

I can't remember a time when I didn't fight for the underdog and tilt at windmills. I stand for the people I love. Growing up in a wealthy family, I thought I could be and do anything. But when I told a family friend and well-known New York investment banker that I wanted to be a multimillionaire philanthropist like him, he laughed at me. As if, 'what does a six-year-old know?'

I've rubbed shoulders with many wealthy, miserable millionaires who, suspicious of *why* they were liked or loved, struggled to trust in their relationships. Money itself does not make us worthy or happy. Yet we love, hate, and judge ourselves because of it. Asking these questions made me a curiosity in my rich world. The investment banker delighted in my perspective and asked how I got to be so wise. I performed at 60% while I hunted the essence of true affluence and how anyone could access it. All I cared about was finding a path to a fair and just world where anyone can be and do anything.

At sixteen, I started volunteer tutoring, including twenty years at the East Harlem School at Exodus House. I was committed to serving my community and deeply ashamed of the inherent advantages my white, wealthy privilege gave me. My discomfort furthered my quest to create affluence for all.

I went through multiple jobs from financial consultant to medical editor, but I was the world's worst employee. I wasn't able to make the kind of impact six-year-old me longed to create. I could see how to empower employees to operate in their zone of genius, communicate better and get better outcomes. I had slim respect for titles, judging people on their hearts and merits, considered in the corporate world as not only unorthodox but a hindrance to efficiency. I fought injustice no matter what it cost me in institutional respect. Without the capacity to help, I was miserable and, ultimately, each time, I had to leave.

The most life-changing event of my life was meeting David Beynon Pena, a talented professional artist, at a church retreat by the Delaware Water Gap in 1992. We laughed at the antics of an eel, about to bite his hand, talked all night and he suggested we watch the sunrise, the moment I fell in love. We discovered David was manic depressive six weeks before we married in 1996. I would do it again. David felt guilty about vacationing if he did not also have a commission or gallery show set up. In Maine, David wanted to paint Owl's Head Lighthouse from the water, so he propped his easel on the seat and, tied to a buoy, painted from a rowboat in Penobscot Bay for a whole day. The attic would fill with paintings as he followed the light, indefatigably, and typically produced two or three alla prima paintings a day.

His dedication to his craft was both inspiring and exasperating for me and he was incredibly versatile, painting portraits, cityscapes, landscapes, flowers and drawings. A brilliant teacher, David could explain complex ideas about art, so they were understandable to anybody. Because of my background, I could have helped him with some of the social cues he was tone-deaf to which got in his way to advancement but, proud, David never let me help. He painted wedding and bar mitzvah events live, while talking to guests and handed off the completed painting at evening's end. David told terrible, long-winded jokes with enthusiasm as I rolled my eyes. He was gregarious, flamboyant and a sharp dresser who prided himself on his hats and vintage glasses. He bought me red roses most weeks and watercolour flower paintings for Valentine's Day. Incredibly attractive to women, I was the only one he saw. He was surprisingly formal and conservative for an artist.

We had twenty-five incredible years together until, in October 2015, David was diagnosed with Stage 4 pancreatic cancer, and our world collapsed. I was suddenly a 24/7 caregiver, faced with losing my husband of twenty years, whose life expectancy was suddenly six weeks to three months. We decided to live fully every second of the time we had left together because one day would be our last. The doctors were very confused by our approach and kept telling him to rest. Why?

By the time David was diagnosed, I had finally discovered the keys to affluence for all and I knew what he needed to do to help him thrive. And thrive David did, and thrive we did. My affluence code work allowed me to design an ecosystem for improving our quality of life. The usual lifespan for a person diagnosed with Stage 4 pancreatic cancer is six weeks to three months, and David lived eleven months. Even the doctors said it was the way we loved and the way we lived.

Everybody has gaps between the life they are living and the one they desire to live. Together, David and I learned the secret of happiness and reached true affluence. True affluence is not about comparing ourselves to others or measuring our worth by the money we do (or don't) make. It's the experience of being enough 'as is.' I discovered that the way people get to 'enough' differs.

Each person has a particular area of focus which matters more to them than any other. Some people need to do their work first. Others need to take care of themselves first. And the rest need to take care of others first. Everybody needs to do all three in a particular order to thrive. How we see the world organically alters how we engage with it, which changes the opportunities we pursue, the decisions we make, the actions we take and being happy and successful.

I realized that people have three core areas of focus which I call lenses. Purpose is the lens whose core focus is work. Love is the lens whose core focus is self-care. Charity is the lens whose core focus is contribution. And business/career, time, relationships, money and health are the five buckets people assess to decide if they are affluent or not. When people don't prioritize *their* way, they struggle or become stressed, broke, burnt out, overwhelmed, ill, injured, or worse...

I am Charity, so I had to put David and our marriage first. We were not going to thrive without support. I had to rely on my community and be bold, clear, and specific about asking my community for what we needed. Shame and reluctance to ask and receive (without obligation) and leverage my community's influence went out the window in the face of our dire need.

I asked:
- for money so I could be a 24/7 caregiver and not be frantic about bills
- for medical professional friends to help me understand data, escalate concerns in the hospital and navigate uncaring systems
- for a self-care ideas list to refuel when I was exhausted (I got 100 self-care tips)
- for connection by FB, phone and email even if I was unable to respond
- for listening and love without judgement or a push to action
- for people who can't handle their own feelings about death to stay away
- for meals and continued visits, especially towards the end
- for friends to show up for David so he could know how loved he truly was
- for appreciation of my public vulnerability on FB
- for seeing me as not just a caregiver (now widow) and not broken
- for audiences to cheer me on at four cabaret shows

- for clients to hire me for Affluence Code consulting, inspired by my speaking out

Self-expression kept me whole. I went public on Facebook and on stage to speak about the three lenses, sang with tears in my eyes, and served with raw truth, inspiration and resources about love, living fully and who we become when we risk it all. I even created a meditation for David and me to fill up with love when we were terrified. So, at the end, he had a roadmap to go out on love.

There are six dynamic archetypes for the Affluence Code, comprised of different orders of the three lenses: Purpose, Love, Charity. The strategies of all three Affluence Code lenses are yours when you are leveraging them in the right order for you. Mine is Charity/Love/Purpose while my husband, David's, was Purpose/Love/Charity. Practically, what that meant for us was that, in times of stress, my bedrock was community while his was work.

Love was David's and my second lens. For us, it was about focusing on ourselves and receiving unapologetically. I discovered that the moment I got crystal clear on my desires, someone provided them. We were given a cuddly blanket, essential oils, food, money, funds for oxygen not covered by insurance and open invitations to participate with others. With appreciation, love and practical support, our families and friends showed up for us at hospitals, in the cancer care centre and at home. We simply received for the sake of receiving without shame or reciprocal obligation.

Purpose lens first, David's core focus was his work. Earning money was so enjoyable for him that he took on multiple jobs. By October 2015, David was working six days a week, and we were paying the price of lost intimacy and resentment in our marriage. The story of our epic love affair was inspiring but, in truth, our marriage was secretly in trouble until he was diagnosed with cancer and we both chose us again.

His 'day job' until May was ushering in the theatre which gave him steady income, structure and work colleagues to joke around with. David taught a beginner drawing class in Summit, NJ which students took more than once because he was so exceptional until he landed in the ER with diabetic ketoacidosis. Losing those jobs hurt him and made him doubt his value.

He painted on-site events, mostly weddings, bar mitzvahs and bat mitzvahs, while talking to the guests, and handed off the finished painting at evening's end. David even took on a watercolour commission of a horse in the last two weeks of his life and happily shared the near-final draft of his Painting Portraits with a Bold Brush book with my Mom four days before he died. 6' 3' tall, he went from 268 pounds to 146 pounds in eleven months as the chemo and cancer took their toll. His doctors told him to stop, just stop. I encouraged him to keep working, prioritizing his painting first. So he did. His biggest struggle was seeing that he mattered when he was no longer able to work so hard, not just for what he did but for who he was. I miss him.

In 2010, working as a medical editor, I asked myself, 'Is this what you were born to do?' The answer was a resounding 'NO!' Over the decades, I started doubting my ability to fulfil my six-year-old dreams. My career trajectory was so seemingly random that it was viewed as failing rather than seeking. I was afraid to engage fully, risk not being enough or be rejected once I allowed myself to be seen.

All the existing solutions were unnecessarily complicated, so I created my own - the Affluence Code. The Affluence Code work provides the ability to be resourceful in any and all circumstances. It's easy to see opportunities when everything is going well but what happens when facing loss, failure and disappointment? Facing David's terminal diagnosis, we lived my work to thrive, instead of merely survive.

David and I became fearless as we walked the line between life and death. I needed community, and he needed to work until the end. It was an extraordinary time of fear, grief, anger, love, and appreciation. We learned more about love in those months than all our previous years together. We talked about the end we wanted, to be alone at home, and so it was. I reassured him that, in a human body, we need breathe and love, so, when he was ready, he could just go out on love. On September 10, 2016, David lay in my arms, took four breaths and passed away. It was one of the most profound and beautiful experiences of my life.

Suddenly, I was a widow with no idea how to be one. People were uncomfortable being around me when I cried. They made wrong assumptions about my needs. I lived in a landscape of grief to despair, seeking a reason to get out of bed every day. Left with a thousand of David's paintings, watercolours and drawings, I am both restarting my consulting work and taking care of David's legacy. I started my BadWidow.com blog in January to open up all those awkward, unspoken conversations, share insights and provide resources for those who have suffered a loss.

I built my business to provide access for others to a fair and just world where anyone can be and do anything. Then David got sick and leveraging my affluence code work got personal. I went from putting myself last to putting myself first. Perhaps you've done this too. When you are ready to thrive and experience true affluence, I am here for you. I know the way.

Reader Notes:

What Are Your Affluence Code Lenses?

- Purpose - focus on taking care of work
- Love - focus on taking care of themselves
- Charity - focus on taking care of others

What's your *first* lens? Can you guess your *second* lens?

To answer questions I have been asked many times; your dynamic archetype does not change. You have access to *all* the superpowers when you honour yours. There is no *best* way, only *your* best way. Wanting Purpose to be your first lens because it looks easier will be painful if Love or Charity are yours. The third lens is only last, not least.

What Are the Dangers of Ignoring Your Affluence Code?
- Stress
- Struggle
- Overwhelm
- Burnout
- Illness
- Injury

Are you experiencing any of these challenges? In what areas of your life?

Where are the gaps between the life you have and the one you want?

Author Bio:

Alison Pena is an Affluence Code consultant, living in NYC, and new widow. She teaches people how to unlock their affluence code from any circumstances and to navigate losses more peacefully and powerfully. Alison Pena's gift is that she sees people truly and stands for them fiercely.

Alison Pena writes for Thrive Global, Medium and her Bad Widow blog. Among others, she has been a guest expert on Entrepreneur on Fire, How to Start Living Show, The Ambitious Entrepreneur, Join Up Dots, Prosperity Place, Social Media Business Hour and Rags to Niches podcasts. Her first book will be published in early 2018.

Client Marina D. says, 'Our work together changed my life. I mean that, sincerely. Because of your commitment to sharing your knowledge and showing up, I have personally seen a transformation in how I care for myself, connect to others, and set (and ACHIEVE) insanely amazing goals that I never dreamed possible. I'm just in awe of how much I continue to learn from you.'

What if doing things *your way* is the shortcut to easy, congruent results?

Connect with Alison:

<u>Websites:</u>
www.AffluenceCode.com
www.BadWidow.com

<u>Social Media</u>:
www.twitter.com/UnlockAffluence
www.linkedin.com/in/alisonpena
www.facebook.com/UnlockingTheAffluenceCode
www.facebook.com/BadWidowWitandWisdom
www.instagram.com/badwidowwisdom

Book a 20-minute call:
www.bit.ly/UnlockAffluenceDiscoveryCall

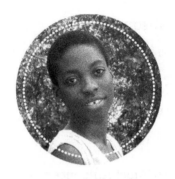

Breaking the Chains
By Lila Simmons

'Owning our story can be hard but not nearly as difficult as spending our lives running from it.' - Brené Brown

I decided when I was 12 years old to marry my first husband ... and I hadn't even met him yet.

Let me explain.

See, my mom was telling me (yet again) about how my dad had cheated on her when she was 8-months pregnant with me, so she dumped his lying, cheating ass. Then, by the time I was 6-months old, my mom was pregnant with my brother, and by the time she was 8-months pregnant with him, his dad had cheated on her...

You see the pattern, right?

Well, my mom didn't, but at age 12, I saw it crystal clear. And at that moment I decided that I was not going to be my mother! I wasn't having a bunch of babies by a bunch of different men, and I wasn't going to keep bouncing from guy to guy without resolving whatever it was in me that created the problems in the first place.

Two short years later, I had the opportunity to put this into practice. My friend invited me to a party. It was more of a get-together. She introduced me to her boyfriend, and then explained to me that he was also dating her best friend. Um...hello polyamory! I thought this arrangement was strange, but if it worked for them, I was happy for them.

Over the next few weeks, the five of us - *Karyn, *Taylor, *Jayven, *Quinton and me - hung out on a very regular basis. At one point, Karyn said to me, 'I think Jayven likes you. You should join us.' I raised my eyebrow. 'Hunny, I don't share,' I said to her. Well, apparently, Jayven *really* liked me because Karyn and Taylor broke up with him and then enthusiastically encouraged me to date him.

For a while, I refused. I just wasn't interested in him romantically. We were friendly, though. Then, one night, we hung out solo because Karyn was out of town and she *insisted* Jayven keep me company while she was gone. He kissed me, and I melted. We began dating.

Not one month into dating and he had a sexual encounter with someone else. I instantly went into 'what is it about me that makes this OK?' Instinctively, I knew that it wasn't about anything being wrong with me. It was about me being attuned to being cheated on.

What I didn't know at the time was that there were generations of infidelity in my family. My grandmother cheated on my grandfather. My uncles cheated on their wives and my aunts cheated on their husbands, except for the ones that didn't. The aunts and uncles who remained faithful, including my mother, were the ones who were betrayed. The healing work that I was doing wasn't just for me. I was healing generations of pain and making sure my own children would have different futures.

Breaking Old Patterns

Determined not to be my mother, I didn't break up with his lying, cheating ass. I started watching Dr Phil & Oprah and reading *everything* I could get my hands on about self-esteem and healthy relationships. My M.O. became read, apply, repeat.

Abusive relationships aren't horrible 100% of the time, or we wouldn't stick around long enough for them to be really abusive. Jayven was charming and romantic. The man could date! He once gave me an experience that started with a limo ride to the local mall where he'd shopped for me at various stores and left gifts. Each store had directions to where my next gift was. Store employees gushed and encouraged me to marry him. If only they knew. And yes, I did marry him. We'll get to that in a bit.

I fell in love with Jayven because he listened to me. There was a time when we genuinely were friends. We hung out together, watched TV, listened to music and laughed. A lot! Being with him made me feel like I wasn't alone or crazy, that is until it didn't.

Every 6-9 months, I would find out he was cheating with yet another person. I would cry, yell, throw fits and then forgive him. Only, it wasn't legitimate forgiveness. Instead, I was burying the hurts on top of each other. After the fight, the apology, and the promise to never do it again, I'd ignore the fact that anything had ever happened in the first place...until it happened again 6-9 months later.

Healing from all of this took years and occurred in layers. In truth, I'm still recovering, but we'll get to that at the end, I promise.

Speaking My Truth

The first thing that I had to do was tell myself the Truth. I took it a bit further and told him the Truth as well. I'm not sure that it was helpful to our marriage, but it was to my Soul. Iyanla Vanzant once said, 'state the facts and tell the truth'. The reality was, I was in love with him. So deeply in love that my face lit up whenever he walked into the room and six years into the relationship, he still gave me butterflies. My Truth was that he was no damn good for me and I told him this. He wasn't sure how to respond which was okay because he didn't need to. Speaking my Truth was my intention; getting a rise out of him was not.

Acceptance was another key to healing for me. It was imperative that I accept him for who he was. During our entire relationship, I was trying to mould him into the man he told me he wanted to be but couldn't because, well, life. Understanding that life could be hard and being an empath, I could literally feel his pain. I made it my mission to help make his life as easy as possible so that he could step up and be the man he envisioned himself to be.

Ladies, this never works! You cannot raise a grown man. Only he can raise himself. If a man is actively healing through therapy, coaching, energy healing or a combination of the above (or other methods), then he's serious about his healing and could be worth the time and energy investment. On the contrary, if all he's doing is complaining about being life's victim, kindly move on if you can. I suggest you seek healing yourself if you're not able to walk away from an unhealthy experience. Seek a therapist or a healing artist like myself who can assist you in resolving the patterns in your subconscious that is attracting that type of person to you. Otherwise, you will continually attract people like that.

My best friend at the time told me to accept him for who he was - a liar and a cheat - or leave him. This was the best advice I'd ever been given. There was something empowering about not being judged for the choice to stay with him. That place of total acceptance was what ultimately allowed me to leave the marriage.

That wasn't an overnight decision, however. Two years and two children later, he fell in love with someone else. He was 30, and she was roughly 22 and a student at the local University. The months leading up to me leaving were full of stress for me. Having no idea that I was pregnant with our 3rd, I was still nursing our middle child. Instead of having a partner to raise our children with, I was home solo with two toddlers, and on the verge of disconnection from our utilities and eviction from our home because we were behind on everything. Meanwhile, he spent nights in her dorm room with her.

This experience was the straw that broke our marriage's back. I called my mother and asked if the offer to take her spare bedroom was still available and being my Mama, she said yes.

For 12.5 years this man had lied to me and repeatedly been unfaithful. I'd been sitting on a gloriously high horse. Living with my mother knocked me square on my butt! My mom spoke negatively about her boyfriend, and because she was choosing to be with him (they weren't even married!), it made my skin crawl. What's more, she didn't communicate with him what was upsetting her. Instead, she talked about him behind his back.

Life as a Mirror

Standing at the kitchen sink listening to my mother rant once again about her long-time boyfriend, Spirit hit me with 'you do that'. I raised an eyebrow (probably literally). 'What do you mean?' I asked the voice inside my head. 'You talk negatively about Jayven all the time'. I could only roll my eyes because I knew God was right.

Two wrongs don't make a right. Jayven lying and cheating on me gave me no right to speak negatively about him, and to him, every chance I got. The difference between my mother and me was that I didn't say anything behind Jayven's back that he wasn't already aware of. My actions were still wrong.

Over the next 16 months, I apologised for where I went wrong in our relationship, and I accepted Jayven's apologies for his part in the breakdown of our marriage. If I'm completely honest with you, I can't say that I forgave him, or even believed his apology. I acted as if I did, however, and when he requested reconciliation, I agreed.

From a very young age, I had an idea of the family I would like to have someday, and it did not include dad living in another state, not raising the minis with me. The most significant part of my healing was letting go of that idea. Over 7 years after he walked out the door, I'm still healing that aspect of this experience.

That idea is why I enthusiastically agreed to reconcile when he asked along with the fact that God had shown me how I'd failed as a wife the first time around. Because I know that if I don't heal something, I'm destined to repeat it, and I was determined to be a better wife this time around; more supportive, kinder, more loving.

Knowing that this man was cheating on me, I got up every morning and made him breakfast and coffee before work. Why? Because that's the type of woman I am. For 13 years, I'd had one foot out of that relationship, and it showed in my words and his actions. Determined to do all of this healing with him, I committed to showing up fully and communicating openly.

What were the results? He left. Yup! He packed his bags and took a job in another state. I asked him to stay and share the house with me. We could have each had a bedroom and raised the minis together, but I assume his pride wouldn't allow him to do this. He told me he was leaving for a job. I'm convinced that had he stayed, he would have found one.

Healing Old Wounds

As I said earlier, his leaving didn't resolve everything. The night before he left, I had an experience that brought me to healing fears of abandonment. We sat on our bed, and he explained to me that he was taking a job in another state. Calmly, I told him why I believed it was not only a bad idea but a choice that would harm our children, as my daughter was already experiencing separation anxiety every time he left for extended periods of time. He listened, then assured me that he had no choice. A lot of excuses later, I said: 'OK, drive safely'.

The miracle in this is that I asked for what I desired. An emotional wound from childhood left me refusing to ask for what I wanted, while simultaneously fearing abandonment to the point of near-paralysis. In the past, I'd begged him not to leave me out of fear of being alone. Begging wasn't me asking for what I desired; it was me desperately grasping at not being abandoned again. That evening, when he left, the abandonment wound healed.

But he was still lying and cheating. Our last month together, he lied about sleeping with two different women. It wasn't until two months after he left that I resolved the lying thing. He decided to have a relationship with a former friend of mine, and when I mentioned it, he denied it. It wasn't an accusation, and I went to him with a very light but direct tone. There was no reason for him to be defensive, yet he was, which is how I knew he was seeing her even before he admitted it.

At the same time that their fling started, I found the source of the lying. I had a belief that men lie. This belief was gifted to me subconsciously by my mother. I had no idea it was in there, but as I was seeking to heal, there it was. I gave my mind examples of men who I believed were honest such as TD Jakes, Joel Osteen and my late father-in-law, therefore replacing the belief that men lie with the Truth that some men are honest. I also demanded that I attract honest men to me.

I cannot say that I've been lied to since. It also appears that the cheating was related to the lying because I have not had an exclusive lover break that exclusivity since my former husband either.

Today, seven and a half years after he left, I'm in the healthiest romantic partnership in which I've ever been. The healing I did wasn't just for me. This healing touched generations. The cheating (and possibly the lying) was present in 90% of my grandparents' children's relationships; they were either cheating on their partners or on the receiving end. Because of the healing I've done, my children get not to have these experiences. They get to see what healthy relationships look like. It's my hope that as you read this, the healing touches you too.

Author Bio:

Lila means Divine laughter or the laughter of the Gods and she is wisdom and giggles on a mission to bring light to the dark places in the world.

Lila is a dedicated mother, a healing artist, practicing multiple modalities from energy healing + mindset work to essential oils + prayer, a bunch of people's best friend and a dynamic story teller.

Connect with Lila:

Facebook: www.facebook.com/lifewithlila
Instagram: @lilaslight

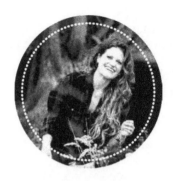

Memoir of a Fearless Love Goddess
By M. J. Robertson

'It's not the absence of fear, it's overcoming it.
Sometimes you've got to blast through and have faith.'
~ Emma Watson

June 5th, 2017. Age 35. Currently living in the UK and travelling *a lot*. It has taken me 35 years to feel into my purpose and to feel good in my own brutally honest, scarred and unapologetic skin.

I'm no longer ashamed of who I am. I no longer feel guilty for being me. I am no longer afraid of speaking up, for having a voice. I no longer fear being seen - whether I am angry, dancing sensually or wearing grubby sweats with no makeup and dishevelled hair. I am no longer afraid to be invisible either.

I am proud of who I am. I've made peace with me. I am thankful for the voice within me, promising sunlight at the end of a dark and thundery storm. I know I am blessed to have a heart full of compassion that dared to be different, and fiercely believed that the world's paradigm could change. I never gave up and I never will. I surrendered my life to a higher power when I was 19 years old, after a series of what I now know people call 'spiritual awakenings', and a whole lot of drunken-drug-induced confusion.

I am now a published author, online entrepreneur and a fearlessly radiant human being. This is my story.

Early Years Memoir

I grew up in a small industrial town called Chatham, Ontario, Canada. Surrounded by a French-speaking farming community, I attended French Catholic School, learning to read, write and recite the Lord's Prayer in French and going home to an English speaking Mom and Dad.

Mom grew up in a well-to-do family, in an even smaller town than Chatham. She was the summer festival queen in high school and had ambitions to be a professional theatrical songstress. She had every ounce of talent and intellect to make this dream a reality. Dad was a hard-working, attractive, practical man who grew up in a traditional household, and whose father was in the RAF. Dad sought a safe and traditional family life. Both of my parents were adopted.

The fairy tale marriage fell apart when I was 5. My parents divorced when I was 6. Mom's mental illness saw her in and out of psychiatric hospitals. I vaguely remember visitations. The dark, wet parking lots Dad brought us to contrasting with the fluorescent lights of the hospital cafeteria.

My sister, three years older than me, protected me and kept my fairy tale alive, playing with me until the pain she was carrying was too much to bear. Our playtime morphed into me running into corners, avoiding eye contact, never being able to say the right thing or dress the right way. My sheer presence had me hiding away in fear, punched into submission and teased when I couldn't hold back the tears.

I was always an introvert and yet, writing down my memories, I can see now why I spent most of my childhood alone. Playing for hours with my dolls, locked away in my bedroom, and disappearing into the woods, the creeks and fields, my aloneness felt safer than company. I'd play by myself for hours and get lost with the neighbourhood dogs and bring home snails and snakes from the nearby creeks. I'd spend a few hours throughout the week with friends, taking trips to the shop to buy candy and attending pool and birthday parties, but I'd always tend to max out with 'friend-time' and need to withdraw into my own inner world.

My mother seemed to respect my solitude and understood something about me that others did not see. As I grew, she encouraged my need for withdrawal, allowing me 'spiritual rest' days as she called them, especially when the pressure of school started to get the better of me. I put a lot of pressure on myself, and always needed to achieve. Even at a young age, I would stress out, have panic attacks and stay up late finishing school reports.

From the age of four, I'd set out my outfit the night before and organise my binders, pens and pencils in an orderly fashion. I remember now, as I settle into my life purpose, being chosen to lead. I won speaking contests, led school performances and from a very young age, teachers told my mother I had a knack for creative writing. Of course, I did forsake it all by the time I hit puberty.

Life was spinning out of control. My sister and I moved away from Chatham to a big new city. We lived with friends of the family, while Mother stayed behind and waited for the house to sell. The drama and turmoil of life and trying to fit in took over, and I succumbed to 'trying to be normal'...whatever the hell that means. By this time I had secretly begun starving myself, exercising obsessively and whenever I got full (which was any time I ate more than an apple), I threw up.

I hated myself and my life. My worth was solely focused on how skinny I was. My value was calculated by how I could match up to the beautiful young women in teen fashion magazines and MTV music videos. I had stacks of *Seventeen, Sassy,* and *Starvation is Sexy* (just kidding, the last one was not a real magazine, but it may as well have been). The hours spent alone playing with my dolls and the trees as a child were replaced with reading these delusional trash mags and watching music videos, fantasising about escaping my world. I believed that if I could only be pretty and skinny enough, I might just make it.

University: The Lonely Years Memoir

Let's just say, I survived high school. After a suicide attempt, I decided to replace the Prozac prescription with self-study and cannabis. I was finally free. I made it. I was accepted into a Canadian Scholar program at the University of British Columbia with an unconditional offer and decided to major in Women's Studies. Even in the world of academia, this subject was ridiculed. 'Why isn't there Man's Studies?' fellow students would quip, as if my field of study was a nuisance to them. I found it fascinating, and of course, I also felt enraged, 'why wasn't I taught this when I was twelve'?!

My awakening had begun, and I was angry - angry at the elitist game of academia, the systematic control of what we call the patriarchy and at myself...because I still just wanted to be skinny and famous so I could save the world and tell all those greedy twats in politics how to properly manage the economy. I wanted to remind people that money is not the answer – *love* is. Argh! The insanity of this world damn near crushed me and my conflicted mind drove me further and deeper into a despairing darkness.

Meanwhile, I was still exercising like a maniac, pushing myself hard to get an acting agent, auditioning for stuff, taking professional dance classes and completing all my study-duties like a good girl. I was still a loner, and eventually, the pull of the 'cool-kid' circle drew me in. I was tired of being a loner and having no friends. It appeared that my few high school friends were having the time of their lives at University so, I started drinking (I was already smoking a lot of cannabis as a regular, self-medicated, loner activity), and eventually, I was offered cocaine and ecstasy. I felt the fear, the propaganda filter in my mind that if I snorted a line of cocaine, I'd end up a junkie, and then a more profound thought, *'but do you want to live in fear of this stuff forever? Try it. But know it is not the answer.'* And that was it - for over half a decade. An awakened, intelligent woman with promise - who spent the majority of her twenties partying and crying and screwing in the shadows.

Rape. Deep self-loathing. Poverty. Aloneness. Chaos. Betrayal. Lies. Is it worth it? Is life worth living? Cause mostly, I wanted to die. I wanted the torment to end. I ran away from my family. Cut all ties. By then I was alone in a foreign country. I'd failed at life. My dreams were shattered. The sparkle of my early awakening was fading with every passing year and my desire to change the world was ripping me apart. It was all a broken, distorted mess.

Yoga Years Memoir

Enter yoga. Three months in India after an abortion because I didn't know who the father was. The end of a six and a half year relationship because I cheated every time I got blackout drunk. In lots of debt. No home. Nearing thirty and *again* pleading with both of my parents to bail me out with whatever they could afford - just to get me some food and pay my rent. My car was on its way to the dump, and I was relying on the generosity of strangers who came to my donation-based yoga classes to buy me food and put a roof over my head. This was *not* how I thought my life was going to turn out.

Any thread of power I thought I had over my life was spinning well and truly out of control. I now call this 'the free fall' phase - once you've surrendered your life to a higher power – and when you stubbornly pursue your ego's projections. Eventually, you hit rock bottom, skid out for a while until you're totally, 100% on your knees and ego-broken.

This 'rock bottom' looks different for different people. For me it was: Friendless. Homeless. Destitute. Three sizes too big and too ashamed to admit defeat to the people who attended my yoga classes. So, even though I'd apparently lost everything and had nothing, I kept practising and teaching yoga.

Yoga was my lifeline - like for real. I made just enough money to buy myself food and offer a kind stranger a measly £35 per week for a room in her house. When the bank letters got threatening, I finally had the breakdown of all my breakdowns. I cried and pleaded with my mother, and she told me I had to face it. This time, instead of just sending me money, she told me to go to the bank and sort it out - like a grown up.

At 29, I realised there were one too many ways I didn't think or act grown up, and it was time to face my many shortcomings. Fess up. Own up to the fact that my life was a mess because I made reckless choices - not because I was a victim of circumstances. I dried my tears, went to the bank, gave myself a serious pep talk and decided I was going to make this 'yoga job' work.

Shortly after that the yoga studio where I worked closed, and I had two choices - go home to Canada and find work while living with either my mom or dad - or take responsibility for my life, meditate like a badass, keep doing yoga and carry on. I chose the latter. Within a month of the yoga studio closing, I had almost 20 private clients and the classes I set up were a hit! They were packed. And, for the first time in my life, I was making money doing something I loved, was passionate about and felt in alignment with my deeper knowing.

I also turned 30 and started writing again. The promise of a better life kicked in and I felt inspired.
Everything was coasting along rather nicely. I was dating a talented, kind and attractive young musician. We eventually moved in together and were supporting one another in living our dreams - learning, growing and talking about how we wanted to make the world a better place. As I observed his discipline and enthusiasm, something in me shifted. I started to feel restless, like there was more.

I'd started blogging, vlogging and was still teaching a lot of yoga. I set up local talks, to share my 'new paradigm' inspiration and insights, which I never planned, just spoke what came through. I never planned a yoga class in my life, either, it just came to me. I'd been accumulating momentum via research and study, in particular, *A Course in Miracles,* and watching a whole load of YouTube videos about the Law of Attraction.

My speaking career began the same year I attended A-fest, aka Awesomeness Fest, which is a four-day gathering of thought leaders, authors, teachers, coaches, healers and some world class inspirational speakers. I was home. Alongside my speaking, I slowed down on the blogging for other sites and focused solely on my own writing with the intent to publish a book. I entitled it *The Path to Paradise* because what was happening to me was nothing short of miraculous. The way my life was transforming in front of my eyes was something that people needed to know. Compared to the suffering I'd been living for 20 years, I felt like I was living in paradise.

I struggled, of course, to validate myself, because so much of it was intuitive. I continued to study and took part in a yearlong alternative energy healing course called Soul Directed Sovereignty, and learned a great deal about energy, soul contracts, collective agreements and something that I now call 'the karmic backlog' which is aligned with the scientific field of study called epigenetics. In short, our DNA is encoded with patterns from our ancestors, and (if you believe in past lives) our own energetic memory bank is acting out unconscious energy patterns from our past lives, hence karma.

So many dots were connecting that my mind was blown on a regular basis, and my life kept getting more astonishing. The book was writing itself.

The Big Leap *Now* Years Memoir

The big leap happened in 2016. I decided I didn't want to be teaching yoga in the same way anymore. I was growing weary of the weekly grind. Seeing people week in week out, making enough money for holidays and nice rented accommodation was not where it was at for me anymore. I knew deep down there was more. I was capable of more and I desired more; more adventure, travel, freedom, impact. I felt burdened and stifled by the yoga community and still felt like an alien in one too many so-called spiritual circles. Everyone talked nice, but it didn't excite me. It felt flat, dull and dense.

While hosting my first surf yoga adventure, I bought a ticket to Bali. When I returned, I ended my relationship with the gorgeous musician, moved out of our charming barn conversion and borrowed £10K from the bank. I went to Portugal, and Morocco, worked with a mentor, and in Bali my first book was written. The original 44 page manuscript of *Path to Paradise* became *The Fearless Life Guide: An All To Love Project* and now supports readers around the world in their spiritual awakening and transformation. It is also the foundational material for the online, donation-based study group called *The Fearless Life Tribe* where I share intuitively almost every day, guided by my soul and a deep burning desire for everyone to be able to transform their lives and see their own loving world.

I've made well over 10K in book sales and Tribe donations. The big leap was worth it, and I'm happier than ever living in the flow, carving my unique path into paradise.

Never-ending Memoir

Just like when I was writing the closing words of *The Fearless Life Guide*, I am now getting teary-eyed with a lump in my throat, because life is so beautiful - just saying those words makes me full-on cry. I've arrived because I am no longer afraid of this world - or anybody in it. How? Because I know that *it is me.* And as I fearlessly continue, guided by my soul and moving to the beat of my own heart, I know that I am safely loved and supported through the darkest of storms to the light, and another sunny day on this glorious, loving Mother we all share, called Earth.

Deep breath. Wipe tears. Go play.

Author Bio:

Molly Jayne Robertson was born in Chatham, Ontario, Canada. She left home after having a series of spontaneous spiritual awakenings while studying at the University of British Columbia in Vancouver. She has been intuitively guided by her intention to create a new paradigm on Earth; the fearless life.

As the founder of All To Love, she is an Inspirational Speaker and author of The Fearless Life Guide: An All To Love Project. She hosts Diving Deep yoga, surf and self-love retreats in tropical destinations throughout the year and regular Fearless Love workshops both online and in sacred locations worldwide. She is a resident yoga and meditation expert at Yeotown, an award winning wellbeing retreat in the UK.

She has been speaking professionally since 2014 and is excited to be touring the UK festival circuit in 2017, speaking at Soul Circus, Wonder Fields and Free Harmony. Molly runs an online private membership group called The Fearless Life Tribe, which supports people in their spiritual transformation. All To Love is a movement dedicated to living fearlessly and pioneering a new, loving and sustainable life on Earth.

Having personally experienced the transformational power of love, it is with a sincere and compassionate heart that she shares her message with the world.

Connect with Molly:

Website: www.alltolove.com

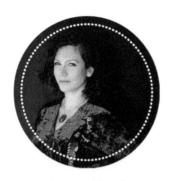

Uncaged
By Harriet Waley-Cohen

'You are the one that possesses the keys to your being.
You carry the passport to your own happiness.'
- Diane von Furstenberg

When I was growing up, I rarely felt enough, certainly not acceptable, likeable or loveable. From my appearance to my achievements, choices, ideas and potential, no matter what *you* saw on the outside, the inside chatter was negative, judging, criticising, measuring me up and making sure I fell short. And even when I achieved, looked great, was praised or told I had a great future, the negative voice inside always took over.

The very first time I remember not feeling good enough was on the school bus aged about six. All the girls were sat up front playing with each other's hair, making braids and ponytails. I have thick, unruly, curly hair that is pretty much un-stylable – and I got some cruel comments that day as no one wanted to play with my hair.

As I got older, I spent a lot of time studying what made the popular girls cool. Was it better to be a high-achiever or was it more attractive to fail? Sporty vs going to nightclubs? Into boys vs not into boys? Every school was different! Each time I switched schools, I would re-invent myself, trying to be the 'cool' girl from the last school, convinced that now I'd cracked it, that everyone would love and accept me, yet somehow still falling short. I needed everyone's approval to feel ok with myself to counter the internal criticism. Each time I wore a new mask, it never worked. Instead, I stepped further and further away from who I was. Those feelings and thoughts of being unacceptable got louder and more persistent. It never occurred to me that me, exactly as I was, was enough.

In my late teens, waif mania hit the fashion scene. Kate Moss was everywhere in the media, with her androgynous, curve-less figure. My natural slim and curvaceous body was now no longer acceptable. I knew for sure something must be wrong with me; none of the clothes in the shops looked good on me. So when an older man who was hanging out with the top models and popstars took an interest in me, I couldn't quite believe it. Finally I had my passport to acceptance...I thought I'd 'arrived'.

Escaping Reality

Having low self-esteem and losing all sense of who I was made the perfect recipe for being taken advantage of. Within a short space of time, the relationship had turned from fun and exciting to abusive and horrendous. I'd become isolated from friends and family; there seemed to be no way out.

Instead of asking for help, I pretended everything was okay and chose to escape the reality of what was going on by saying 'yes' to every drink and drug that the older, glamorous crowd offered. By the time I was 21 years old, what had been a coping mechanism dressed up as fun had turned on me big time; the darkness of addiction had taken hold. My body weight plummeted by a third within two months, and I started to become a prisoner of my mind. By this time my boyfriend was casually supplying drugs to friends, so there was a near constant supply at home.

Fast forward to the age of 25; I knew things had to change radically or I was going to die. People I'd partied with were dying, and any fun had long since gone. Instead of nightclubs, famous people and gorgeous dresses I now spent my days hiding in my flat with the boyfriend, barely eating, getting wasted and thinking desperate thoughts in my head, feeling confused about the way life was turning out. This continued day in, day out, often calling in sick to work and unsurprisingly, my career was a non-starter. The relationship had become increasingly toxic over the years; he mistreated me on every level, emotionally, financially, physically and beyond (a cycle of abuse he continued in subsequent relationships).

In hindsight, it's easy to see that when you treat yourself like crap and allow others to as well, you will have little value for yourself. What had been the solution to my low self-esteem had become the very thing destroying me and feeding my inner critic with powerful fuel.

Deciding to Change

I left that relationship in 2001 and thought being free from him would mean that *I* was free. Except I wasn't. The illness of addiction still caged me. By the following summer I'd had enough; there had to be a way out, yet I couldn't see it. I had no idea who to talk to or what to do. Then, a nasty horse riding accident left me lying flat in a hospital bed for several days, allowing me space to finally make a life-altering realisation that things had to change, big time. At the time, I was in excruciating pain and struggling to walk on crutches. However, I determined that things could only get better.

Once I was home from the hospital, healing slowly, I learned the hard way that deciding to change in itself wasn't enough to actually change...and a visit from an old friend saw me picking up drugs again. I knew then that I couldn't create change on my own; I needed help.

By chance, a couple of days later, a documentary was aired on television about the effect of addiction on young women ,and the trauma they experience in the midst of it, all very similar to what I'd encountered. Seeing other women going through it was like having a mirror held up, being shaken awake, punched in the stomach and stabbed in the heart at the same time. There was a helpline to call at the end, and I rang it immediately, crying, scared yet relieved. Maybe the cage didn't need to be locked forever, and there was a way out?

I asked for help and started to attend 12 step meetings. These changed my life radically. From the very first meeting, I had a glimmer of hope, and a much-needed sense of belonging. As time went on, life took on new meaning, and glimpses of happiness started to shine through. I rediscovered what it was like to laugh, to wake up without a crushing sense of self-hatred, frustration and dread. I had an impending sense of ok instead of an impending sense of doom!

Healing from the Inside

The meetings helped me to understand what I'd been through, to stop blaming myself for being a bad person, and to see that what I was suffering from was an illness, not a moral issue. Relationships with others - and myself - healed. Vitally, I started to learn how to change my behavioural patterns, discovering a spiritual way of being that gave me total peace of mind about everything and enabled me to turn off the critical chatter in my head. I fixed myself from the inside out, rather than trying to change what felt wrong on the inside with stuff on the outside. I loved the friendships, support system, sense of belonging and peace of mind that arrived. It felt, and still does, like the best gift and best decision I've ever made.

When I reached a year sober, I decided to heal my body on a deep level and had some sessions with a nutritional expert. He showed me how to eat in a way that worked with my body and the foods to avoid that I reacted badly to. I embarked on a cleanse that cleared my liver and kidneys of all toxins. My allergies disappeared within days, and my eczema cleared up as the toxins left. This process of learning to honour my body through food was very healing, and my body started to trust me again. I discovered on a deep level that self-trust and self-esteem are actions and not states of mind, that how we treat ourselves on every level sends a signal to us about our value. The door of the cage felt more open than it ever had before!

Stepping Out of the Cage

I wish I could say it has been plain sailing all the way since then, that the last 15 years have been nothing but success, love, health and happiness. However, there have been more cages to flee, more freedom to find and clarity to emerge. I have learnt more about myself, my values and what's important to me, stepping into alignment with my newfound knowledge before exploring another part of myself still bound and caged.

First I released myself from the financial world. My career took off brilliantly after I sobered up and within a few years I reached management level. However, after my first son was born, I knew with total clarity that my career, with its long hours and stressful deadline driven environment, was incompatible with being the kind of mother I desired to be. So, I left and devoted several years almost entirely to motherhood.

At the same time, I sought professional help for some of the trauma that I had been through during the addiction years, freeing myself from the past, allowing myself to live in the present and create a beautiful future.

It became apparent after about eight years of marriage that my husband and I weren't compatible with each other. We had very different values and were both unhappy. Unfortunately, this manifested as infidelity and various unkind behaviours from the side of my now ex-husband. By the time I was ten years sober, I knew that I had to release myself from the relationship, for the health and sanity of both of us, and our two children. It was a very emotional, hard, long considered decision, but one that has ultimately proven to be very positive for all of us. We now have a good relationship, and co-parent effectively with mutual respect.

It was after leaving my marriage that I started to look towards creating a business where I would devote my energy to inspiring and empowering others to change their lives, while also being the kind of mother that is present when it matters for my children. I trained as a coach and as a speaker. The coaching training filled me with enthusiasm and excitement and came naturally. The speaker training, on the other hand, was a much bigger challenge – I arrived at my first session nervous, nauseous and petrified, afraid to say so much as my name out loud.

However, something beautiful started to happen during my speaker training. I discovered a vital principle for being a successful speaker: from vulnerability comes power, connection and impact. Finally, I could release myself from all shame of the past, letting go of the fear of judgement from others. It was time to embrace telling my whole story, and show who I truly was to inspire and empower others.

What has followed from this shift has been phenomenal. The minute I started getting honest on stage about my journey, letting audiences see me 'naked' – no mask or pretence or need to be liked - and shared my story with truth and authenticity, the impact went through the roof. Bookings started to flood in, coaching clients appeared in abundance, and I began to see my mission – to make sure every women knows how to feel deeply, truly fabulous about herself - come alive in front of my eyes.

Now I am a sought-after speaker and coach working in the personal development, corporate and educational spheres. I get invited to tell my story to teenage girls at schools, inspiring them to honour themselves, to have courage and resilience. This feels like such a privilege and the beautiful messages that I've received from some of the girls have had me in floods of tears.

The power of releasing the need for approval and feeling ok about myself has been truly life-changing, not only for me, but also the thousands who have heard me speak and the dozens whose lives I have helped change as a coach.

Additionally, knowing myself and honouring myself on every level has become the foundation of which so much happiness and change has happened, and this has rippled out far beyond me as I show others how to do the same. I treat myself with nothing but love and know with absolute clarity what I am bringing to the world, why and how. Living my life with love, grace and clarity is fabulous; I am finally unstoppable, unbreakable and free.

Reader Notes:

What would happen if you let go of needing external approval to feel ok about yourself?

What if instead, you focused on getting to know yourself and honoured that in every area of life?

Take a moment to imagine what becoming in total partnership with yourself would be like. How would your life look? How would you feel?

Author Bio:

Harriet Waley-Cohen is a highly sought-after speaker and coach, and mother of two gorgeous boys and a cockerpoo called Fizzy.

In her speaking and coaching, Harriet empowers women to be in total partnership with themselves in every area of life. Women who work with Harriet find themselves no longer overwhelmed, on the edge of burnout, full of self-doubt and coping with destructive habits; instead, they become truly confident, full of self-esteem, balanced, emotionally and physically well, fulfilled and successful.

Harriet has a B.Sc. in Psychology and is a certified coach with both the Institute for Integrative Nutrition, New York and One of Many in the UK. Before training as a coach and speaker, Harriet had already dedicated significant love and energy to being a volunteer mentor to young women with drug and alcohol issues for over a decade. Having been through multiple transformations, including leaving banking for entrepreneurship, ending an unhealthy marriage and going on to flourish, and being over 15 years in recovery from addictions, Harriet is ideally placed to understand the kind of love, support, guidance and tools that it takes to make deep-rooted life changes that stick.

Connect with Harriet:

Website: www.harrietwaleycohen.com

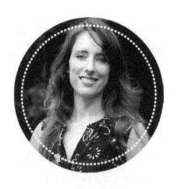

Don't Should on Yourself

By Tamsin Astor

'Self-care is never a selfish act - it is simply good stewardship of the only gift I have, the gift I was put on earth to offer others. Anytime we can listen to true self and give the care it requires, we do it not only for ourselves, but for the many others whose lives we touch.'

- Parker J. Palmer

Good girl. Ugh. That's what I was, on many levels. I loaded the dishwasher. I turned in my homework and got 3 'A's in my A-levels. I said please and thank you. I held the door open for seniors. I wrote thank you notes. I brushed and flossed my teeth. I married the first guy I fell in love with and had his mother over for Sunday lunch.

But there was a part of me that rebelled against this deeply. As a young girl, it manifested in what I wore (crazy enough that my mother would sometimes walk 100 yards behind me), the colour of my hair, the music I listened to, the musicians and much older men I dated.

When it came time to get a real job, after college graduation, the thought of getting up at 6 am every day and putting on an ironed shirt, jumping on the train with thousands of others to work in an office block, with no natural light, made me feel ill. Hmm. How to rebel, but not fuck up my life too much?

I decided to persuade my parents that I needed to discover life's true purpose and the only way to do that would be by spending six months in India. But then my Undergraduate project advisor, Patrick, took me aside. Patrick - a tall, skinny, bicycle-riding vegetarian - said that my data was sexy (his words) and warranted a deeper dive. Had I considered doing a PhD?

Over a bottle of red wine that he carefully warmed under his office lights, as the sparkly night of London opened up behind us, we concocted a plan. I applied and started a PhD program in the fall of 1998. Perfection I thought. I could wear whatever I wanted, work whenever I wanted, spend hours every day tangling with ideas (sapiosexual is definitely a box I check in my online dating profile), read articles and stick electrodes in people's heads. I was working towards becoming a Professor - a real, proper job!

Phew. There again I was managing to balance my inner rebel, my inner badass with being a good girl on the outside, making sure that I was doing what I *should* do! By 25 years old I had been awarded my PhD, owned a house and married my first love. Life seemed pretty fucking sweet.

We moved from London to St Louis, Missouri, and did Post-Doctoral fellowships. I was starting to doubt whether academia was for me - the politics, the peer-reviewing process to get published, the fight for grant money to do meaningful research, the way academics turned their noses up at teaching. In fact, the goal was to do as little teaching as possible to show your prowess (thus proving your ability to teach little and have more time for research). So, just before I turned 30 when my second son was born, I quit.

We moved to Cleveland, Ohio and I realised that being a stay-at-home-mom was SO. NOT. MY. THING. I loved to breastfeed. I loved to wear my babies. I loved to take a weekly mom-and-me class. But, OMG I craved a bigger stage. I yearned for an intellectual world beyond my family that was engaging and pushed me to challenge skill sets that were not being met by motherhood. The *shoulds* of trying to be a stay at home mother were getting the better of me and I knew I had to break free.

I trained as a yoga teacher. I trained to teach kids and teachers how to use yoga and meditation in classrooms. I taught people to be yoga teachers. Somehow none of this was ever quite enough. I still felt caged, somehow, like I was doing what I *should* do, but not what I really wanted or needed to do. This feeling was exacerbated by a number of massive events that shook me and ultimately shattered the cage I had been living in and made me realize that creating a life built on '*shoulds*' doesn't prepare you for the (inevitable) collapse.

The first involved my younger son.

My two-year-old son started throwing up one summer. Every fifteen minutes for 6 hours. Worried about dehydration, I took him to the ER. Stomach flu they said. A month later, the same thing happened again. Again the ER said nothing's wrong. We became concerned and asked his pediatrician to order tests.

Thursday, September 4th, 2008, 11pm I was stroking his hair, as he was finally asleep after 6 hours of testing in the ER. The nurse came into the room and said: 'the pediatric oncologist wants to talk to you.' I stood up and left the room and a sweet, grey-haired man came up to me, looked me in the eyes and said, 'we need to run one more test, but I am convinced your son has cancer.' Just breathe, I thought. In and out. That's all you need to do right now, is breathe.

The next day the tests confirmed it and he had the surgery. Watching your child come out of general anaesthesia is truly frightening - their skin is grey, their breathing unnatural, their body too still, too heavy. As he came around, I could see the confusion in his eyes. He had a nasogastric line coming out of his nose, an epidural in his spine, an IV in his arm, a catheter, a drainage line in his abdomen and a wound that stretched from his belly button to his waist.

The next year involved more surgeries, two rounds of chemotherapy, a suspected return of cancer. The waiting. The appointments. The holding him down so they could draw his blood, or put in IVs or numb his port for the chemotherapy drugs. The constant weigh-ins, the weight loss (25% of his body weight), the hair loss ('mama there are spiders in my mouth' - the clumps of hair that would collect as he slept).

This experience woke me up. I started studying and learning and doing a lot of self-work. I intuitively knew that I needed to find a way of engaging that stopped me from living a life of '*shoulds.*' I needed to figure out how to start looking after myself, so when events happened that were out of my control - er, hello, life - I had the skills to process, digest, manage and come out stronger.

It was the only way to live and was something that I had to embody if I wanted to make it through this experience with my mind-body intact and with the learning that I knew I needed to take on.

I had to be happy NOW, for this moment, this moment was my life. I couldn't live as if I would be happy when.... I had to find that peace and joy now, because who knew how long it would last? I had to prioritize my self-care and create a more stable inner world.

As we re-drew our family unit, by having a third child, and learned not to focus on every single sickness, my husband struggled. He was trying to get tenure, and the powers that be were making it hard. The stresses resulted in my developing insomnia, food allergies, IBS-like symptoms and a commitment to the *shoulds*. I *should* make all my kids food from organic farmer's market produce. I *should* weigh this much. I *should* have yoga biceps/triceps. I *should* have shaved legs. These *shoulds* took a toll on me.

Western doctors suggested I suppress my symptoms with pills and perhaps a few tests and more pills. It did not sit well with me. I did not like being told I *should* take something to suppress my experience!
So, I went down the path of Ayurveda (*ayus* - life, *veda* - science) - the sister science to yoga. The focus was on creating healthy daily rituals, such as regular bedtimes,

mealtimes, meditation, self-massage. It was tough for me. I had spent the last decade putting everyone else's needs before my own! It felt selfish and indulgent, but I knew I did not want to become a sanitised, medicated shell. I knew I had to face myself - every part - and learn how to nourish myself if I was going to figure out how to navigate this thing called life.

I trained in Ayurveda because I felt its fantastic effects on my life along with Yoga Health Coach training, in this Ayurvedic model. I trained to be an Executive Coach, developing my social and emotional intelligence and corporate leadership coaching skills. I realised that this was my thing. It was my jam. I had finally found work that resonated with all parts of me. By Fall of 2013, I officially launched my business.

Fuck yes, I thought. *It's all coming together again!*

Or so I thought.

The cage that had reformed following my son's survival from cancer was weak and shattered again in 2014.

My cousin-like-a-brother died of leukaemia in January of 2014, when we were both 37. The fucking c-word was back with a vengeance. As I started to digest this event, things took a bad turn in my marriage.

In July 2014 we went on our family vacation and on day three my then husband walked out leaving me to explain his disappearance to our kids, his family, his cousins, and friends. By that point, he had walked out on the marriage three times. This time I was done with the '*I should keep this marriage going for my kids' sake*'. I knew that this cage was truly shattered and my inner badass, the Phoenix, was ready to rise out of the ashes. This marriage was finished.

Over the next 18 months as we navigated the divorce, I took an approach to my healing that lead me to delve deep into my own experience so that I could also help others.

Every week I wrote a blog detailing the shitstorm that was my life. But rather than sinking into woe-is-me, I presented the nasty stuff and talked about how I was handling it. Because, you know, my mind is like fucking Manhattan real estate and I am not going to give it up to someone who doesn't deserve it.

Suddenly people were responding to my writing differently. I wasn't saying meditate because it's good for you. I was saying - *meditate because when your heart is breaking as your four-year-old is weeping on your lap about how much she misses daddy's girlfriend, it will help you and allow you the space to heal, and enable you to be the kind of mother you want to be.*

Eat kale because it's got Vitamin K, is high in antioxidants and will lower your cholesterol, became *eat kale because the majority of the feel-good hormone serotonin is in your intestines, so if you want to feel good, don't eat crap food!*

Life evolved, the divorce was finalized. We bought houses two blocks apart from each other and worked on communicating about our kids, for their sake. We rebuilt our relationship as co-parents and now, we co-parent peacefully and celebrate our children's successes together, such as celebrating our teenage son's recent successful black belt test for Tae Kwon Do.

I built my business, I worked with clients. I wrote a book, submitted it to a publisher and got a three-book deal. Life was sweet. I felt like I was starting to live life on my own terms. The *shoulds* were starting to get under control.

Breathe.
Be present.
Be in the now.
Just breathe.

And then, again, my feet were pulled from underneath me.

During the winter of 2017, I experienced a number of deep personal boundary-breaking interactions with people in my life which fit in with the cultural tide of the #metoo movement and once again shook my cage. These related to my being out and open, both personally and online and vulnerable about myself and my life and people assuming they knew me and projecting their desires and obsessions onto me.

Breathe.
Be present.
Be in the now.
Just breathe.

I withdrew and reflected and determined not to let the projections of unhinged people determine how I wanted to live my life. People will always lie, create drama, project their fantasies and try to manipulate and control others. The key is not to let these people change how I live my life.

And so, following another cage-shattering experience, through the power of the self-care habits I have developed, I have again risen to create my life on my terms.

Each time I have fallen, I have learned how to get up faster, by caring for myself in the ways that I know work for me. This all circles back to the *shoulds*. When I live by the *shoulds*, life is harder because my inner and outer worlds are not aligned. When I live on my terms, caring for myself and prioritizing my needs whilst nurturing that which is important and vital to me, I thrive.

I am living a fully uncaged life. And it's *so. damn. liberating.*

I work hard with my clients. I write and speak and teach. I collect my kids from school, travel with them during their holidays, and I spend my time doing what I want - yoga, walking my dog, cooking, reading, listening to live music. I stoke my fire, my light and fulfill my life's purpose to shine so that I can help busy people organise themselves, so they have time for what they want and need *and* time for fun. The path hasn't been easy, yet here I am, being who I was meant to be *and* being the best goddamn mother, friend, daughter, sister and lover I can be.

Reader Notes:

It's not selfish to prioritize your self-care, your joys and pleasures. It's so easy to put the needs of others before our own. As a parent or primary caregiver, *think of yourself as the lighthouse who shines on others. Nourish your light.*

What is *one* thing can you do for yourself, every day?

What can you celebrate about yourself? Look for things to be grateful for!

a) Grab a piece of paper. Write down everything you do every day - literally everything, including washing, peeing, shopping, cooking, going to meetings, commuting, teaching etc.

b) Then group everything into three columns – things you LOVE, TOLERATE and HATE.

Do the math – what percentage of your time are you doing things you *love*? Then reflect and use these two main tools to create a shift:

Change your mindset. For example, are there things that you have to do, but you HATE or TOLERATE them? For example, do you TOLERATE bathroom times? How about getting new towels, painting the bathroom, scheduling enough time that you enjoy it?

Delegate it to someone else or delete it.

The purpose here is to add more to the LOVE column!

Author Bio::

Tamsin Astor, PhD
Chief Habit Scientist

I help busy professionals organize themselves so they have time for what they need & want, and time for fun. I am your Chief Habit Scientist, wrangling your habits around sleep, exercise & eating through a lens of mindfulness & relationship management. We make tens of thousands of decisions every day, so if we can create connections between the habits that serve us well, thus reducing the number of choices we make, we free up lots of time. This irony - creating routines to create freedom is what I love to help people activate in their lives! I draw skills from my extensive training (PhD, RYT500, Certified Living Ayurveda, Certified Executive Coach and Certified Yoga Health Coach) and background (research, teaching, parenting a child with cancer, a child with ADHD, coaching) to guide clients through change related to their careers, relationships, physical health, and emotional health.

Connect with Tamsin:

Website: www.TamsinAstor.com
Facebook: www.facebook.com/TamsinAstor

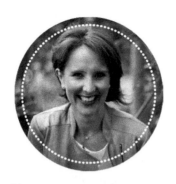

All You Need is Love
By Ella-Louise Woodhouse

*'Perfectionism is a self-destructive and addictive belief
system that fuels this primary thought: If I look perfect,
and do everything perfectly, I can avoid or minimise the
painful feelings of shame, judgement and blame'*
~ Brené Brown

My heart and soul felt like it was splattered all over the floor
and yet I felt completely numb. Two and a half years
together, a future of dreams - business, home, family - all
over in the blink of an eye. All because I had pushed.

I was 30 and having to start over... again. It was a recurrent
pattern; fall in love, feet first, and then at the point where
most women would be dreaming of diamonds and settling

down, I would turn, my frustration and anger mounting to the point of explosion. I would push them away, pushing so hard that it broke.

'My heart sinks as I walk towards the front door as I don't know what sort of mood you're going to be in', he said. It was like a dagger through my heart, and I felt the guilt and rejection crushing down on my chest so heavily I could barely breathe, but this was pretty much the pattern.

Why did I always have to break relationships? Push them before they jumped so devastation couldn't come out of the blue and catch me unawares? So I wouldn't be surprised by the rejection? So I could say to myself 'I told you so' and prove to myself that I didn't deserve to be happy?

Family Life

My Mum and Dad divorced when I was one year old, a wise move on my Mum's part although they kept a good relationship for years. My dad was mostly a good dad, in the early days when I could still be sat on a stool in the corner of the pub with a cola and packet of pork scratchings. He taught me how to ride a bike, cook, enjoy gardening, and revelled in embarrassing me with his ministry of funny walks in the supermarket.

Once my stepmother came on the scene, however, things changed drastically. My father lost any backbone he ever had, and she began running the show, which meant as little association as possible with my family, and maximum opportunity to belittle me. Dad's relationship with my mum broke down while my stepmother's contempt for me grew. She appeared to take pleasure in either ignoring me or throwing condescending remarks my way. The kind of comments that would typically go over the head of a seven, eight, nine, 10-year old, but they hit me, each and every one. It was only my Dad's head that these nasty quips appeared to soar over; him wanting a quiet life while I was left feeling sick and scared, and never sure what mood she was going to be in... sound familiar?

I remember one Sunday night after being dropped off home falling in the doorway in tears, so relieved to be back with my mum, stepdad and siblings. I offloaded all the horrible things that had been said to me that weekend. My mum had reached her limit and said she was going to confront my dad. I was petrified – the thought of upsetting him was too much. What would my stepmother do to me if she knew I had snitched? I begged mum not to say anything; I was terrified that she'd ignore my pleas.

She did not raise the issue with my father until just after my 30th birthday when a little skit of my stepmother's threatened to ruin the party. After a frank and open letter was sent to my dad, intercepted by my stepmother, and a pack of lies being sent back by her, my parents never spoke again.

I grew up with my younger sister and two brothers, my mum and stepdad. Our childhood at home was a happy one and full of love, no arguments or crossed-words that I can remember. So when as a young teenager I overheard my stepdad whispering on the phone one night, I chose to ignore the lurch of my stomach. This was one of my first lessons in trusting your inner wisdom as a few months later it transpired that he had been having an affair.

Losing Control

It was around the same time that I was studying for my exams. I had recently gone on the contraceptive pill, and having never counted a calorie in my life, had gained fourteen pounds in just one week of taking the hormone. Coupled with the fact that I was no longer a straight-A student and the increasingly asphyxiating feeling of losing control of my whole life, I began to diet. Nothing seemed to work, and with the hormonal imbalance in me, it was unlikely to.

I tried not eating, restricting myself to one slice of toast and an apple all day... but after a short time, I realised I was hungry and faint, and that wasn't conducive to trying to keep up at school, so I progressed to binging and purging. I would stuff my face and then stick fingers down my throat to get rid of it all. I was useless at first, walking away before the point of being sick... but before long, it was an addiction. An adrenaline rush of control. I couldn't sleep until I had done it just one more time, to make sure nothing was left inside of me. My skin was blotchy, I was bloated, and yet no one knew. I felt like I was rebelling against the world, but was also desperate for someone to notice, take me in their arms and help me find a way out of the maze.

Having developed ME/Chronic Fatigue Syndrome in my late teens (a result of screwing with my body), I left school due to ill health and began working in a restaurant. Over the next five years, two more relationships were ruined thanks to the constant battle of wills inside my head. One side of my mind told me I was fat and unworthy of any relationship, while the other more sensible side knew that I was being irrational.

I remember sitting for family feasts at my boyfriend's parents and running to the toilet in tears, shaking with fear. I feared being expected to eat it. I feared gorging myself and facing more self-loathing. And I feared breaking down in front of everyone and having to tell them what I loser I was. It was the loneliest time of my life, being so scared of who I was and what people might think of me. But how could I expect anyone to stick by me if I couldn't even admit to myself what I was doing was wrong? So the fear, the anxiety, the disgust built up inside and all I could do to protect myself was to create a shield to deflect the emotion - the anger, hatred, resentment - onto those closest to me. Many happy family get-togethers were ruined because I was so wrapped up in my own self-loathing and obsession.

It was a vicious cycle; whenever anyone close to me was in a less than pleasant mood, my lack of self-worth told me it must be me, I must be the issue... so I would redirect their mood back at them 10-fold, to show that I didn't care. And so the cycle escalated until the relationship broke.

After the Christmas when my boyfriend of two and a half years could not take it anymore and ended up having a cliché affair with his on-stage panto princess, I decided leaving the country was the only option. Running away from the heartache (because that shit can't follow you, right?!), I landed a job as an entertainer in Mallorca and then Crete. I met amazing people and had the best summer of my life. In the sun, everything seemed better and working 15 hour days, six days a week in the public eye was a sure-fire way to keep a fake smile on your face. I thought I was happy but was knocked sideways when my body issues took hold halfway through the season, and I began struggling with what I saw in my reflection versus keeping my demons in check. Nevertheless, I soon fell in love again, this time with a colleague from Germany, and we saw the season to a close together before both moving back to Berlin.

History on Repeat

Another fresh start; new job, amazing new people and, aside from an initial headache trying to pick up the lingo, I felt sturdy on my feet. Then in a flash, everything seemed to turn. My boyfriend was sent away to do his National Service, a dear friend in the UK had a severe heart attack and my stepdad had another affair and left for good, tearing our family apart. It was all too much, and I went to work one day and collapsed to my knees, sobbing. I remember thinking I should get up, but couldn't. I was stuck to the floor, rocking, and howling. A full-on breakdown. Antidepressants and my friends out there got me through, but it was apparent I needed to come home. So I did and started again.

It wasn't long before I was in a very wrong and very turbulent relationship. The next couple of years were destructive, with anger and frustration building up on both sides. He wanted to control me, and I didn't have the strength to fight, so I lost who I was and became a shadow of my former self, afraid to speak up or have an opinion. He did make me seek help for my eating disorder, and I went through Cognitive Behavioural Therapy, but the deep-rooted emotions continued bubbling away, threatening to erupt at any moment.

After a long, drawn-out break-up of our engagement, relationship and possessions, I enjoyed the high life for about two minutes before falling for the next guy. He was the complete opposite to the last (they always were). He was younger, laid-back with youthful ideals, and I took on a motherly role, which was not his wish but what I thought I had to be.

We were happy for the standard two-year quota, and I finally saw myself settling down, but as time went on, I began to resent him. Resent the role I had created for myself. I wanted him to take charge and look after me, but I treated him like a child, and he behaved like one. I controlled everything about our life together. I could not allow him his freedom, as unless I was in control, how could I be sure we were having a good time? That we were in love? The necessity to plan and monitor how happy we were was so overwhelming that it made us both dreadfully unhappy, and I broke it.

Wearing a Mask

While I started to deal with the heartbreak, a life lived in fear of being seen as needy or weak meant I had a volcano of trapped emotion bubbling away under the surface, with little mini-explosions every now and again. To the outside world, I appeared frenzied and hectic. I remember my neighbour asking me one day, 'are you ok? You seem a little manic?' Looking back, I was! My eyes were wide; I regularly had the shakes. I was working as many hours as I could fit into a week (over 80 some weeks), just to make sure I had no time to think, no time to reflect, no time to feel lonely... no time to deal with the dis-ease my life was in.

I was anxious going out in a group. I put on a front, laughed ever so slightly too loud and was always conscious of people watching me and judging whether I was having a good time. But I was scared they would see through the façade and see me for the boring person I thought I was!

During this time I set up my first entertainment act with a couple of friends. It all started as a bit of fun but quickly grew and, not having run a business before or laid down ground rules at the beginning, the cracks began to show. I was a perfectionist and wouldn't stand for less. As we took on more girls and problems arose, I took it as a personal slight, and a lack of respect for me, instead of accepting responsibility for not managing the group better. I was fumbling around trying to find my way and learn how to lead, and I did not see the resentment building up in the others' eyes. It came to a head out of the blue one day, and after a barrage of abuse directed at me, I lost a colleague and best friend. Just a few weeks later my boyfriend left for the same reason as the rest... I made him miserable with my authoritarian approach to a partnership... I was still the common denominator!

So it was all about control. Controlling my destiny, my happiness, and the experiences of people around me. If I wasn't in control then what on earth would happen? Things would fall apart and catch me unawares. If I let go, then who was I? If I relaxed and enjoyed the experience of life, then people might see the real me, and not like me!

Emotional Freedom

I discovered Emotional Freedom Technique through my mum who is also a practitioner. She had done it for years, but I hadn't been open to it until it was the right time for me. Rather like acupuncture without the needles, it focuses on trapped emotion causing a blockage in our energy flow. Throughout our lives, we experience emotional spikes on a daily basis - some small acute incidents, some chronic issues that weigh down on our psyche and knock us off balance. By tapping specific meridian points, we can release that pent-up emotion and allow the energy to flow smoothly again through our system. You don't need to believe it because it works anyway and the great thing is, you can do it anywhere and anytime. The person next to you doesn't even need to know you are doing it!

I have tapped, and continue to do so, for so many specific memories and general feelings of emotion that have built up over the years. It is amazing how by dropping baggage, you can feel the weight lifting and your energy brightening.

The adage 'you have to love yourself before anyone else can love you' is so true. I always used to think that 'loving yourself' meant arrogance but it doesn't. What it means is knowing your worth, knowing you are deserving of happiness, knowing you are a good person... and by believing in that you open yourself up to endless opportunities for happiness. So many amazing things have happened in the last five years; love, marriage, a daughter, travel, business success... peace!

Don't get me wrong, we all have our off days, but now I tap. I tap and ask myself 'what is this feeling about?' I acknowledge my thoughts, the guilt/frustration/self-pity/blah-blah-blah, but these thoughts are fleeting, and I watch them pass by. What helps move these storms along is by being *grateful* for what I have. There is so much to be grateful for when we are open and aware, and it can bring us back from lurking in the shadows, to see the beauty in any situation.

A wise lady, Marina Pearson, said to me recently, 'life is happening, whether you are in control or not, life is going on... so you can sit back and enjoy the ride'. That resonated with me as for so many years set on controlling speed, direction, passengers on-board, stopping points etc. has meant missed experiences. I make time to enjoy precious moments now, and I enjoy expressing love to others. It makes you feel good, and it sure makes the other person feel good too! What difference could we make to the world if we slowed down enough to enjoy the ride and shared our love with others around us?

Reader Notes:

Take a moment to reflect on the following:

1) What are you trying to control in your life? What would happen if you let go of the reins and enjoyed the ride?
2) Are you true to yourself when out in a group? Do you open up enough to let people see and connect with the real you? What would happen if you were just 'you'?
3) What ten things are you grateful for today? What have you seen, heard, smelt, experienced that lifted your soul, even for a second?

This is all about allowing yourself a better way of life for your future.

Connect with Ella:

Website: www.head2health.com

Faith

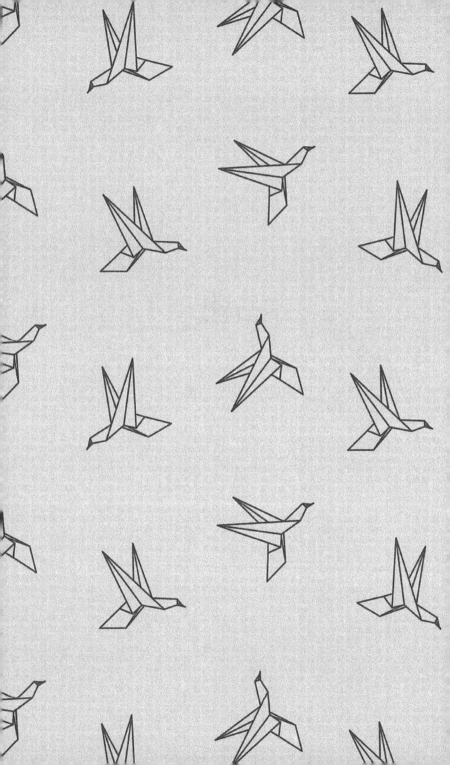

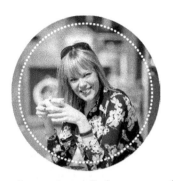

The Dark Side of the Workplace
By Josie Copsey

'You can never leave footprints that last if you are always walking on tiptoe.' ~ Leymah Gbowee

What was your childhood dream? What did you want to be when you 'grew up'?

Even as a child I was ambitious, hungry to progress and develop my skills. I was the model student; studious, well-behaved and keen to build a successful career. As a high-achiever leaping into full-time employment, employers would see the potential in my soul and determination in my eyes, feeding my insatiable appetite for personal growth and development with ongoing training and career progression.

By the age of 25, I had reached my career goal, securing a middle management position and delivering a training service to over 2500 employees. My career was soaring. To the outside world I was flying high and going places. Yet behind closed doors my personal life was falling apart.

An ectopic pregnancy at 25 almost cost me my life. And to make matters worse my then boyfriend had finished our relationship only two days previously. With the trauma of hospitalisation and loss I needed something to lift me out of the darkness. I turned to the only thing that I knew, the one thing that proved my success when all else was failing: work. It's often said that when one area of your life suffers, another soars. In my case this was true. Despite my personal tragedy, by the age of 30 I was promoted again and now sat on a leadership team with significant responsibility within a tough culture organisation. I thrived on the pressure and accountability. I knew the difference I could make to the company, the impact I had *already* made. I craved the acknowledgement and acclaim that I deserved. Progression was mine for the taking.

I was an established change professional, confident in my abilities and potential. So, I decided to take the plunge and move into rough waters, stepping away from the comfort and security of a permanent role and into the uncertainty of the more lucrative contracting.

Landing my first contract as the only female in a boardroom of twelve, I was put through my paces. In a male dominated environment I *had* to prove myself. And I did. Yet after taking enough kickings, criticism and back-handed compliments, I decided that it wasn't for me and when I handed in my notice, four of my male peers followed me – I'd paved the way! Though that's not the story I want to share with you in this chapter, this was the start of things to come. Fast forward a few years and I joined a heavily male dominated team in a FTSE 100 company. You know the kind. Inappropriate comments disguised as office banter. Raging testosterone as the men competed with their peers. This was nothing unusual in my line of work. However, a couple of the new male leads - the ring leader of whom was my boss - were clearly on a mission to prove themselves. And what better way to do it than to belittle the woman; this is when the professional bullying started.

Despite being brought into the business *because of* my expertise, these particular colleagues repeatedly undermined me, consistently (and very audibly with the intention to humiliate) told me how to do my job, and ensured that I knew my place in not only the organisation but the world. I was continuously reminded of my remit and ordered not to have any discussions with senior leaders without them being present or made aware that such meetings were taking place. I was made to feel that I was unimportant, that my opinions and skills weren't of value and that I didn't matter. I was the weak and feeble little woman that would never be taken seriously and who had to earn her right to be heard. Ignored, snubbed and on many occasions, ostracised.

No one else in the team experienced this. I was being singled out. And perhaps no coincidence that I was the only woman.

Sitting on the same bank of desks as them, I was appalled at how they would speak about women, namely their wives. Often crude. Always disrespectful. These poor women were oblivious to what their beloved husbands/partners were saying about them behind their back. Maybe they did this to wind me up and get a reaction. Maybe they really *were* that misogynistic. Who knows? I didn't bite and just sat there listening, smiling politely, daring not to break or show emotion in front of them, instead focusing on doing the best job I could to earn their trust and respect somehow.

Little by little I slipped further into low self-esteem as I pushed increasingly to prove that I was competent, that I was capable, yet their words and dismissiveness continued to eat away at me, chipping at my confidence.

After much deliberation following a long weekend away from the toxicity, I returned to work and gave notice to leave. The look of relief that swept over my boss's face said it all. With an agreed end date in 4 weeks, he asked if I could ensure a thorough handover with detailed notes, along with my extensive catalogue of documentation. This was a big ask.

Starting my notes the following day, he called me into a meeting after lunch to check in on how I was doing. After only 20-minutes he told me to pack up my stuff and leave. Immediately.

I was shocked. Stunned. I hadn't done anything to warrant or justify this behavior. Clearing my desk and acknowledging the very few colleagues I'd built working relationships with I left the office feeling numb, appalled, embarrassed and pretty damn small.

The feeling of being pushed out, *forced* out, left a bitter taste in my mouth. A part of me felt relieved. I no longer had to endure the mental hell, *torture*, anymore. Yet I felt lost. Confused. My heart was telling me one thing, that this was for the best, that it had happened for a reason. But my head was telling me that I'd failed, it was my fault, that despite all my efforts and achievements perhaps I wasn't as good or successful as I'd thought.

As I drove home, the egoic emptiness grew – what was I going to do with my life? Who was I without a career? Some days later, the emotions changed into anger. Then worthiness. Or lack of. For the first time in my successful career, I felt stripped of my ability to do a good job. Was I unlikeable? Why did they pick on me? What did I do wrong? Unanswerable questions raced through my mind for days, over and over, as I tried to make sense of it all. Feeling lost and unsure of what I was going to do, I retreated to a converted barn in the beautiful Kent countryside, a place that will always be magical to me. I had the barn to myself and switched off from the outside world – my phone, friends, family and even the TV!

It was here that my real journey began. No distractions allowed me the stillness I needed to re-discover who I was. Over three days I took walks in nature, journalled, meditated and underwent Reiki. I unearthed answers that were already within me but had lain buried. I started to understand where it had all gone wrong.

With tears streaming down my face, I grieved the ambitious girl in her childhood who wanted to succeed, the twentysomething who lost her baby and boyfriend at the same time and now the woman in her 30's who had sold her soul to someone else's dream. No wonder I didn't recognise myself; I wasn't me anymore. This person was an amalgamation of everybody else, *their* dreams, *their* success, *their* expectations. I carried a little piece of someone I'd met to keep a status, a job or gain promotion.

I realised that my desire to succeed came from a place of longing - for acceptance, to prove that I *could* do it, to meet the high standards that were set throughout my school career, the times that I'd gotten praise and recognition for working hard and doing a good job. I'd attached my level of success to my level of self-worth. And failure had never been an option.

Through my journalling I started to list my strengths, the things I wanted in my life, along with those I didn't. I began to add things, places, interests that made me happy. I started to ponder how I could get more of this into my world, the things that brought me joy rather than pain. A plan was forming, a new dawn was rising. Goals made, actions and timelines in place, I took back control of my life; this girl was going to make it happen.

I'd like to say it was straightforward and I came back from my retreat to live the most beautiful life ever. But real life doesn't work like that. And bills still needed to be paid. Despite my awakening I still had financial responsibilities. Though this time I had the comfort of self-belief....and a plan to see me through!

Taking another contract in the corporate world, I stepped down from my previous positions of authority - everything that I had worked so hard for - and took a role without the burden and responsibility. It felt liberating not to attend senior leadership meetings or make critical decisions or even to take the stress and pressure of work home with me. Having the extra headspace enabled me to focus on my personal development outside of work. I enrolled in courses that interested and fascinated me – Reiki, massage, nutrition and life coaching. I developed a whole new hunger for learning and growth. My spiritual awareness grew. Whereas before external validation quenched my thirst, this time I ventured inwards and followed my soul's desires and evolution, regardless of the outcome and reward.

Over 18 months, my entire life had changed. I moved to another county after buying my first house, my dream house that I had asked for during my retreat. A new circle of like-minded souls had entered my life and my relationships with my family and friends were improving. Finally, I got the opportunity to start up a new business, integrating both my passion, my career and my spirituality, helping others to quit selling their soul in both their work and life.

You don't have to be a victim of bullying. You *can* be true to yourself without compromising your unique gifts and identity. The world is crying out for more women to bring their true essence to the workplace and I'm here to help you do exactly that.

Reader Notes:

Happiness is an inside job and while I've worked through my identity and career path, life is still an ongoing evolution. Every day presents new obstacles and opportunities to learn, should we choose. My biggest lesson has been to trust your heart, or gut as we commonly say. When something feels 'off', even if we cannot rationalise why, there's always a reason. Trust this and you won't go wrong.

Author Bio:

Josie Copsey, Life Change Expert, Speaker, Mentor and founder of www.aeracuralifecoaching.co.uk helps people stop selling their soul to the wrong job, environment or career and start living the life that they desire.

Working for 17 years in senior transformational roles for large corporate businesses and experiencing corporate bullying first hand, Josie is passionate about revolutionising the working world by helping individuals to be true to themselves without compromising their unique identity and authentic self.

Josie's mission is to change the dynamics of the working world, and see the rise of individuals following their heart and applying their talents to their desired career, whilst enjoying their life.

Connect with Josie:

Visit www.aeracuralifecoaching.co.uk to access Josie's highly successful life change plan, which keeps even the toughest procrastinators on track with their goals.

.

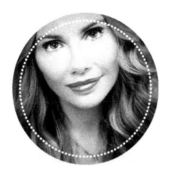

Coming out of the Kundalini Closet
By Lisa Bardell

'You are a light that cannot darken. You are a soul that shines through. You are the eternal amid the moment. You are awakening. You are love' ~ Creig Crippen

In summer 2016 my spiritual Awakening ramped up ferociously in intensity, to the point I lost total control of my physical body. My reality, my way of living daily, changed forever. No longer could I choose to dip my toe into the spiritual waters and retreat when it was convenient. I was on a ride with no end and no way of getting off. And for a while, it was terrifying. Otherworldly, bonkers, and completely isolating. I felt uncomfortable sharing my experience with people because I was right in the midst of a Kundalini Awakening Process, producing symptoms so bizarre they felt demonic at times. I was scared people would think I was psychotic, possessed or both, and that they wouldn't believe me.

So I stayed within the safety of the closet, behind closed doors.

My hope with sharing my story is that you will not do the same if this happens to you because connection, communication and quality information is what you need. I will share some resources that helped me, and they may serve to guide you along your path of evolution.

From Divine Blessing to a Curse

One sunny day in August 2016, after the Kundalini Process had been showing up through me for about a month, it all got too much. It went from feeling like a divine blessing to a curse in the space of a morning. What I know now, is that's precisely what is supposed to happen; you're not meant to cruise through your Awakening comfortably.

What you're meant to do is relinquish the 'I've got this', say goodbye to the illusion of control and fucking surrender. Big time surrender. To be okay with not knowing what the hell is going to happen to your body or your life moment to moment and relaxing into true, deep faith. Faith and trust that you are being divinely held, guided and healed. Faith that the process is in itself the most love you could ever be graced with receiving. Faith that your human equipment is being redesigned and upgraded so that you can radiate more light into the world. And faith that no matter what comes your way, it is happening for you, not to you.

The other side of surrender lies beauty, bliss, magic and miracles. But before it comes panic, shame and utter chaos. I had started the day bursting with bliss and joy, so high-vibe that my human vessel could barely contain the intense energy. Every cell in my body felt like it was about to rupture with rapture. It felt like a force blasting through my consciousness, rising up to my crown chakra and cracking it open. The energy in my head was producing what I call cosmic tinnitus, the mother of all tinnitus with the sounds of the entire cosmos in my head. I felt like I was on the verge of blacking out. Fear was starting to kick in.

I wanted to get outside to the park, and I knew I needed to be on the grass with my shoes off to earth some of this manic energy. I just hoped it would pass.

For about a month before, I had been experiencing spontaneous body movements. They started off gently at first, like tai chi, and had been progressing into more dynamic postures, yoga asanas, mudras and body locks. The technical terms for these are 'spontaneous Kundalini Kriyas'. In the world of the Kundalini Awakening, they are just another-day-at-the-office kind of thing, all part of the process to clear blockages of stuck low vibe energy, and release what you need to let go of to expand your capacity for higher and higher energy frequencies. They became my new normal.

Until this particular summer's day, I'd mainly experienced them in the morning or at night when I was doing my daily practices of energy clearing, alignment, meditations and mantras. But this day was different. Once I got outside and started walking to the park, I could feel this energy of movement within, more physically and dynamically. It was an undulating and unpredictable movement, which was making me feel quite seasick. I had to concentrate on walking, the inner momentum was unsteadying and balancing felt like an effort.

When I got to the park, I sat down, and my arms were starting to move, dancing and flowing out to the sides, fully stretched. It felt good to let them move freely; no-one was around. While normal behind closed doors, I'd never experienced it like this in public. It felt new and odd. Gradually the inner motion and the outer motion got stronger, and the movements wilder. I could force my arms to stay relatively still, but I couldn't stop my upper body from moving. I decided I needed to talk to someone I trusted. This would be the first conversation I'd had about what I was experiencing. When my friend picked up the phone, it was a relief to speak. I told her about how these movements had started, and what was happening. Our humour took over for a while, and we both saw the funny side; I was able to giggle at myself and at how utterly bonkers this all sounded. But beneath the surface, I could hear her concern. It was clear to us both that this was an unpredictable process, and I had no idea where it was all going next. Our call was a welcome respite, but my body had been moving the whole time.

I thought eating might help with grounding, and maybe the normality of a coffee shop would stop me focussing on the movements and calm my uneasy fear of what was going to become of me.

In the coffee shop, it did not go well. While managing to keep my arms still, my convulsing upper body movements were getting more extreme. I could feel my panic at the thought that my life was changing beyond all recognition. Would I have to explain this to 'normal' people? Would they believe me? Would I be sectioned and put on medication? Could I see clients, friends, and run my business? Or would I just have to hide away on a spiritual retreat and just hope it calmed down? I'd had such a beautiful, blessed month with the process and now it was turning. This vulnerability and doubt is what I'd read about. I was so foolish to think I would escape it. I berated myself for being such an idiot.

Fighting Through the Fear

I decided I needed solitude in my office, which was a five minute walk away. That walk felt like an hour. Everything was escalating, the panic ramping up the effects of the Kundalini energy and I now felt like I was being thrust around by an angry ocean's worth of power. Just like standing in a wild sea and trying to walk out to shore, I was being pulled down to the earth, over to the sides and up in the air as if being knocked by a wave. It was impossible for me to walk because if both feet were not rooted to the ground, I would be knocked over. As I walked painfully slowly through the town, my ego still trying desperately to appear normal, I dreaded making a spectacle of myself or being thrust into the air in a demonic way. I dreaded losing consciousness and requiring medical attention.

The cosmic tinnitus felt otherworldly. I feared being hospitalised and getting stuck in the system. I feared for my spiritual safety. And I felt utterly, uniquely, freakishly alone in the world, trapped and isolated in a surreal nightmare. I felt totally powerless and lost.

When I eventually got back to the safety of my office, the body movements went off the scale. But there was no sense of release or relief for me. Usually, I would relax into the asanas, and the 'routines' would have a beginning and end point and a kind of symmetry to them. Now I was just flailing around. Upright, upside side, back bending, trembling, all fuelled by what felt like utter panic. I needed expert advice, but I was too on edge to do my research.

In tears, I called a Kundalini yoga teacher I'd been messaging. She was not an expert on Kundalini Awakening and had not experienced anything like what I described, but she did say I must not get afraid because when you mix fear with Kundalini, it is extremely dangerous!! I'll never forget her Brazilian accent telling me this in a slow, ominous tone. *Holy crap! WTF was I supposed to do?!*

In the next ten minutes, she saved my sanity (and possibly my life). Having someone to talk to made a huge difference, and she guided me through a grounding visualisation where I was sat on the floor and imagining roots growing from my root chakra, deep down into the earth, grounding and releasing the energy.

I was calming down. And so were the movements. I needed to take this much more seriously; I was too far down the rabbit hole to go back now, and I needed help for the future.

Surrendering to the Divine

I found some mentors, good quality information and proper support on my path of spiritual evolution. I realised it was time to fully surrender to the Kundalini and to trust her Divine Feminine energy to heal me emotionally, physically and karmically. That's what she was here to do for me. Any resistance or fear would slow that inevitable process down, or ensure it became a rollercoaster ride.

It didn't. I surrendered and trusted.

What followed that August day was what I call a fortnight of fragility. I felt like an alien trying to pretend I knew how everything worked. For the first time in my adult life (apart from a few fleeting days here and there) I felt unsure of myself and crippled with self-doubt, wracked with self-loathing and complete paranoia about everything and everyone in my life. I was shaky and petrified that something terrible was going to happen.

It culminated in a dark night which I spent awake, talking out loud to myself, loving and praising myself like my own biggest fan. Talking myself up for hours on end seemed to be the only way to direct consciousness and lift me up. I awoke feeling as though I'd broken through something huge. I reflected on the previous few weeks and realised that I'd released many emotions, most of which I otherwise hadn't had conscious access to.

I had been on an enforced ban of any spiritual practice, spiritual reading, meditation, energy clearing, and mantra. Anything that plugged me into source came off the menu until my physiology and neurology had done more clearing, processing and was strong enough to integrate this new up-levelled energy.

Developing a Daily Practise

I now felt ready. And with the help of my research and mentors, I developed a powerful daily system to help keep me aligned, on track, aware of my stories and equipped to clear and release old programs, patterns, habits, traumas and emotional imprints as and when I become aware of them. This has been an incredibly fascinating journey for me, and my thirst for exploring it and honouring all aspects of my soul's evolution has never diluted since.

My daily practice is kinesiology based, which I'm convinced has eased my path immensely. I use it to ask my higher consciousness what my blocks and resistance are, what or who in my experience they relate to, what is causing any physical symptoms, or which energetic cords of attachment with people I need to release. I release specifically and thoroughly using a mantra, and then I always get confirmation from the kinesiology that I have indeed released these. Only at this point do I align and embody the highest possible frequencies that I have the capacity for. Bringing these in through a clear channel feels incredible and sets me up for love, grace and bliss throughout my day. The spontaneous Kriyas have taken on a life of their own; I merely relax and stay fully present to their guidance. Most times I can stop them. Where it's very difficult or impossible to stop them is if I'm in group workshops, sound immersions, group ceremonies, or anything spiritual where I'm connected to source. I decided to get out and connect with others, and that was the beginning of me stepping out of the Kundalini closet.

Most important for me is that the Kriyas and the Kundalini process itself (which is still in its early stages) has brought me to full body bliss which sometimes results in spontaneous orgasms!! The Kriyas can sometimes be very muscular, producing inner vibration – hence the orgasms.

My Awakening Journey

I would never rewind to my pre-Kundalini years. On reflection, I'd been following the textbook awakening path. Before my first activation in 2014, I experienced a rush of sexual energy releasing from my root chakra, powering up through my spine and into my heart chakra where it felt like it exploded. At the time I thought I was dying. It was like a steam train of energy bursting out of my heart centre, and my ribs felt like they were going to smash apart. But before what I now know to have been a breakthrough, I was experiencing a breakdown.

I had lived for over two adult decades with partying and

alcohol being my prime motivation in life and my way of avoiding facing childhood trauma.

By age 41 I was drinking three-quarters of a bottle of gin each night, and that was me taking it steady. I had risen to the top of my fashion career at speed. I exited the business as a board level director of a global company after 16 years in the industry in which I started out as a shop assistant. I was jaded and bored and wanted to return to my passion so trained to become a therapist. In the short break that I took between the two, my world and material identity came crashing down, as a series of concurrent and unpredictable financial crises catapulted me into significant debt and uncertainty. I wanted a quick fix. Little did I know that this was a vital stage of what was to become my Awakening. It was also what I needed to bring me to my knees and force my hand into surrender to faith; I was left with no other choice!

I have learned way more on this journey than I can cover here, and it is bringing magic to my client work in many ways. I live with grace and presence now, which feels more deeply embodied with each week that passes.

Reader Notes:

Below are some key points and resources for you to explore:

1/ There are many types of Awakening; the Kundalini is the rarest, most relentless and the only kind which blasts through from the root chakra. This forces you to address and release all lower energies and imprints held in the lower chakras. Other Awakenings are all top down, from higher chakras.

2/ The Kundalini Awakening Process is designed to clear all blocks and resistance from this lifetime, previous lifetimes, and anything passed to you from your ancestral timelines. It does this to expand your capacity for higher frequencies with the ultimate aim being Enlightenment.

3/ Any practice that can help you to routinely enquire on and clear what is coming up for you, such as kinesiology, will help enormously with this process. A daily routine of self-work and top quality self-care, nutrition and hydration are pretty much essential.

4/ Grounding visualisations and being outside without shoes can help if the energies get overwhelming. Stop all spiritual practice for a while, do mundane things. You will never be sent more than you can handle.

5/ Surrender to the process; you are blessed with it for your soul's highest evolution in this lifetime. Do not wish it away or resist it; all fear creates more extreme symptoms.

6/ Mentors and information will help. I've heard it said that a Kundalini Awakening is impossible to navigate alone. I would agree.

Resources:

Books:

The Spiritual Awakening Guide - Mary Mueller Shutan
Awakening Kundalini - Lawrence Edwards PhD
he Awakening Guide: A Companion for the Inward Journey - Bonnie L Greenwell

YouTube:

https://www.youtube.com/user/FlowingWakefulness

Author Bio:

Lisa Bardell is a Transformational Coach, Therapist and Shamanic Energy Healer. Her signature one to one program for women, Alchemy, facilitates a total transformation in clients over twenty two weeks.

Having surrendered to the spontaneous channeled movements, yoga asanas and mudhras which first started to come through her during a Kundalini Awakening in 2016, these divinely guided expressions evolved into her precise work as a Shamanic Practitioner, following training in 2017.

Throughout 2017, Lisa's work in her private coaching practices in London & Cheshire, shifted emphasis towards Intuitive Energy Medicine, yet she still draws heavily on her training in Clinical Hypnotherapy, NLP & Psychology.

2017 saw the birthing of Lisa's retreat brand, Inner Radiance, which she offers in collaboration with fellow healer & coach Rebecca Ann Wilson.

Their one day events and healing retreats are held regularly in Manchester & London, with longer retreats planned for 2019 in Bali & Ibiza.

Lisa's debut book, *Shine Brighter* will be published in 2018 on Amazon.

Connect with Lisa:

Website: lisabardellcoaching.co.uk
Email: info@lisabardellcoaching.co.uk
Facebook: facebook.com/lisabardellcoaching &
Facebook.com/innerradianceevents

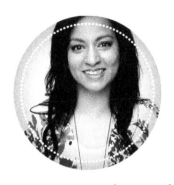

Stepping into the Dark
By Angelique von Löbbecke

'In order for the light to shine so brightly, the darkness must be present' ~ Francis Bacon

I have always been afraid of the dark.

To me, the monster under the bed, the clothes hanging on the closed door mimicking a person, the blackness of the forest and the vastness of space seemed too real.

Having experienced extreme trauma in my early childhood and adulthood, I knew that we as humans could carry an excessive amount of darkness within us. Sometimes untapped, sometimes embraced with a seeing eye, sometimes right in your face.

One of the challenges in accepting the gifts in my journey of becoming a healer was the ability to see this specific quality of darkness, in everyone. To me, it did not make sense. Why would I, who has heard the call to help and serve others, see this particular part of a human being and *only* this part?

Around me and on the internet people would be all 'love and light' and 'Namaste' while I could hardly stand to go outdoors because of the unwanted and unsolicited information pouring into my heart, mind and soul. It took me a while to learn why this was essential. Why this was crucial to learn how and why people heal and how even the experiences in my childhood attributed to this understanding.

'All streets lead to Rome' they say. In my case, all roads lead to one point or crossroad. Allow me to take you on a journey.

The Darkness

Preying on the unsuspecting.
Lingering for an opportunity to conquer and devour.
Hiding in the shadows.

The pain and isolation were very real.

Unlike other kids I had no interest in going for night walks in the forest during field trips or to scare myself to death and find it funny because I could run away.

That was my everyday life as a kid and young adult already. I had learned that I could not trust others. In fact, I did not even trust myself.

I began questioning myself and even the religion I had grown up with. Why is this happening? Why me? Why is there no divine intervention?

Somehow I had managed to stay sane and whole.
Was this the divine intervention? A blessing from God?
I was puzzled...

Every Sunday and every other day I would pray: 'Please God - let me find a place where somebody cares for me. Please make this stop. Please help me.'

But the situation did not change. I tried to bargain with God, tried to make a deal. I made sure I was a 'good girl' and obeyed even if the orders did not make sense to me. During this time I found a place where I was whole. Unharmed. Undisturbed. And this place was inside of me.

Psychologically you would probably call this dissociation, the way your mind shields you from the things happening to you by catapulting you elsewhere, keeping you sane. Later I found out that in shamanism this particular place is called the seat of the soul – and I had found it by accident out of pure necessity or remembering.

Being the late bloomer that I was, it did not occur to me that anybody would show interest in me. Sad, but true, I thought I was ugly.

So when a guy, whom I'll call B, showed up when I was 17 there was not the slightest resistance on my side. I jumped right into the relationship without a safety net. Did I see the signs? Maybe.

He showered me with affection, time, presence and love. Picked me up from school. Escorted me home. Called in several times a day. And I was soaking it up like a wilting flower.

At the time I wasn't familiar with the concept of narcissist and empath. I did not see it coming.

Fast forward two years and my father had to pick me up after my boyfriend had almost killed me. I'd attempted to end his life to save my own, an experience that left me shell-shocked.

We went to Goa, India where my grandmother lived, and for weeks I sat on the beach staring at the rolling sea while the waves, sea salt and sand carried my pain, tears and devastation away. I had left my safe place inside of me, only to find my own darkness.

The Exploration

After recovering mentally, emotionally, physically and spiritually from this episode of my life, I realised that I did have power, over myself *and* my path.

My pain had shown me that I could come out on the other side. That I was resilient. I was very determined, independent and had built a fortress around my heart.

Boys came and went, friendships bloomed and expired, but I just went my way.

There was always quite some drama, and dancing around the edge of what was possible and appropriate held huge fascination with me. My journal harboured lyrics like 'I wear my sunglasses at night', 'dancing with tears in my eyes' and 'your telephone keeps ringing while you're dancing in the rain'. I danced like a mad woman until my feet were bleeding and the morning sun was high up in the sky, took up any job which offered some adventure and travelled around Europe.

Until one day I was head-hunted from college by a TV station to become a TV host and journalist. This was my chance to start afresh and shed my old identity. I moved to Berlin and reinvented myself. The opportunity to start over with nobody knowing me was liberating. Berlin, my new home, never sleeping, never tired, swallowed me and I adjusted my sails and screamed: More! *Give me more*!

The Skyfall

I wanted more, and I got more. Deciding I was ready for love and life without a safety belt, leaning into trust, love and authentic connection became my priority. After all, I was fearless, right? The man, who would later become my husband, conquered my heart and managed to make me open my fortress, doors and windows too. However, the more I opened up, the more information flooded in, most of it unpleasant. Jealousy, doubts, uncertainty. The job, so sought after and glamorous, became a strain on my energy and health but I couldn't see a way out.

An accident turned me and my whole world upside down. After resisting the call for a couple of years, the universe made it unmistakably clear that I was literally on the wrong path and put a car in front me as a dead end, catapulting me and my motorcycle across the road.

The Purge aka The Weight of the World

The darkness, my familiar friend, sneaked up on me. After my awakening, triggered by my accident, my senses were heightened. What was once invisible was plain to see in broad daylight, mocking my sanity.

'Dear Universe, I got your memo...' I affirmed. 'I will face my inner darkness if that means I can conquer it and walk on this new path for the greatest good of humanity'.

So the unpacking of the inner boxes started, in the room where I had locked everything away. The pain. The hurt. The trauma. The violence. The memories. The more boxes I unpacked, the more the feeling of fringing on the edges occurred. The sight of everyone else's darkness did not help either. It was eating away from the outside, while the unpacking of the boxes de-stabilised my inner world. This room inside of me wasn't a cupboard as I had estimated, it was an endless corridor. Box after box after box, never-ending.

You probably don't have to be a psychic or Einstein to assume what happened next: depression and burnout rolled over me. Nietzsche was a smart guy: 'When you stare into the abyss, the abyss stares back at you'.

Was this the price I had to pay? After three decades wasn't that a bit unfair? That I would fail myself by trying to heal? By trying to walk a new path wherever that might lead me? Wasn't that like flying to Mars only to find out you can never return because you miscalculated the fuel?

Again I found myself, this time at the edge of a lake, staring at the water for months and weeks, while the waves, the whispering of the reeds, the howling of the wolves in the forest, carried my pain with me, trying to induce me with courage and conviction.

The ducklings hatched. Watching them grow, day by day, and watching their parents love and care for them while the sun warmed my skin and the birds began to circle in flight, made me believe in love again. In life. In the ability to overcome. I re-evaluated my situation, how far I had come, what I had lost and gained along the way and made a decision there and then: enough is enough.

The darkness, once my enemy, became my friend, or let's just say we acknowledged each other's presence.

While I would probably not jump up in excitement if you asked me for a night walk through the forest today, I realise that we all have all parts in us: the ability to love *and* to fear. Being connected as well as being separated from what nourishes and fuels us.

Separation is an illusion if we are willing to see both sides of what is presented right in front of us.

While I had cursed the hurt others inflicted on me, I could now see how this was also an opportunity to heal and how these occasions shaped me into the woman I am today, able to see the ugliest parts of humanity yet still holding space and light to heal.

The Unknown

The heart is a wild thing. What it wants today might be of no interest tomorrow. But when we desperately desire something we perceive that we cannot have, we question why.

Is it our subconscious? Is it not safe? Do we not want it enough? Should we do more, less, nothing at all? Has our past imprinted our being to a default state where the one thing that would bring us closure, bring us healing, is the one thing that eludes us?

Here it does not matter if what we want is true love, a new job, ultimate happiness or shiny, long hair. Sometimes all we need is just the last nose-length.

Our belief shapes our experience to some extent. If somewhere deep down you think you should have kissed Roger at the party back then, instead of Rob, your relationship with Rob will always be tethered. If you believe that you are worthy and capable of loving, you will probably meet The One and live happily ever after.

But the last ounce, the nose-length, is not your belief, more your ability and willingness to trust the unknown. To trust the process. 'You cannot discover new oceans unless you have the courage to lose sight of the shore', said Andre Gide.

In my case, I was clinging to my old life as a glamorous journalist wanting a new path and unconditional love without giving up the safety of the fortress of my heart and the perceived security of my job. That did not go too well. Only when I trusted the process, embraced even the ugliest and darkest parts of myself and jumped without a safety net that I got a taste of what I longed for.

Is it uncomfortable? I will not lie, most of the time it is. Does it hurt? Probably.

This analogy, recited by one of my teachers, Sarah Petruno, helped me to embrace the process: 'Imagine you are in a flock of crows. You do crow stuff, hang out with them, you are a crow after all. One day, you notice that you are not a crow but a young swan: Your feathers are grey and already turning whitish, but they are certainly not black. So first, you still hang out with the crows, who are saying, they are cool with you being a swan, you are their friend after all. But they are not. You are clumsy, growing bigger and soon you don't feel like doing crow stuff all the time, you start doing swan stuff. You oscillate in-between of the two worlds, while the crows wonder why you are into swan stuff all of a sudden. The solution is not to keep pretending you are a crow but to embrace that you are a swan. Seek out other swans, do swan stuff. Come back and do crow stuff every now and then if you like. You are all birds after all.'

Additionally, life has taught me another lesson: healing and progress occur in cycles. We grow and then shrink or retreat a bit. We grow and retreat again.

As an Aries this is not a familiar concept for me as I was accustomed to going head first into everything, but like the moon and our menses we women roll best with the flow, which might be different depending on which (healing) phase you are in.

Today I am occasionally still processing the changes my personal life has taken (and is still taking) yet enjoying the ability to help others grow past their obstacles as I have grown past most of mine.

Does it take determination? Yes.
Does it take willpower? Sometimes.
Do you need faith? You sure do.

No matter what challenges you face and what you've been through, I can assure you: you *can* do it.

Don't bend, *lean* in.

I have seen it, almost all: the good, the bad, the drama and trauma, betrayal, inexplicable pain, cruelty. And it has lead me to see that there is something inside of ourselves, a place where you are whole and free, healthy and happy. There is also something outside of us, a higher force, source if you will, that can help us bring light to the darkest corners of ourselves so that we can overcome anything and everything.

If I can do it – you can too!

And if not, take my hand: I will sing disco tunes and light you along the way.

Reader Notes:

<u>Action steps to break a pattern</u>:

The Unknown does not feel safe to our mind, especially our subconscious.
Chose one topic where you feel you have been steering back and forth.

Set a timer for 10 minutes and journal how it would feel to be on 'the other side'.

How would you feel, what would you do, how would your life change?

Explore.

The more you familiarize yourself with the unknown, the easier it will get to do the actual steps to get you there.

Repeat the same process and feel into: Why wouldn't you want change?

Sometimes the reasons are very irrational and by bringing them to light you will make yourself consciously aware of your choices.

Author Bio:

Angelique works as a healer and mentor and helps female creatives and soulpreneurs to discover their true power and expression by helping them connect to their innate healing and intuitive abilities, exploring uncharted territory in their emotional world and psyche so that they can live the fulfilled, joyful life they truly desire.

Angelique is based in Berlin, Germany where she lives with her husband Alex and their dog Amy.

Fun facts: likes dragons, crossbows, crystal, glitter and driving fast.

Connect with Angélique:

Website: www.angeliquevonloebbecke.com

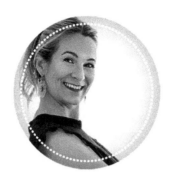

Finding Your Light
By Audrey Michèle

'We are not human beings having a spiritual experience. We are spiritual beings having a human experience' ~ *Pierre Teilhard de Chardin.*

In the summer of 2001, I was about to turn 26. I had everything I wanted, and I was to everyone in my world what they desired me to be, the latter probably being my greatest success! Even before I graduated from the University of Amsterdam, after four successful years studying Communications Sciences, I was hired for the job I'd been dreaming of.

You know what is said about the Vision Board, right? You cut pictures of what you desire to have in your life, paste it on a board, look at it every day, and *voila,* everything you want will be yours. Well, that is what I'd been doing to get that job without even knowing about the concept of the Vision Board: I saw the advertisement for Ormit for the first time inside a student magazine. I immediately loved the description and *knew* that this would be perfect for me after graduation. I cut the page and put it on my desk. For the next six months, I looked at it every single day. And the closer I got to graduation, the more I could feel the excitement and certainty of joining this company growing within me.

So there I was, in Amsterdam, about to proudly finish a Master of Science within four years. With classes and study materials given in Dutch and English, neither of which is my mother tongue, you bet I was proud! Or maybe I should say that in the present tense... because even if it was already 16 years ago, it is still one of my proudest accomplishments.

I mean, I was 19 years old when I went from France to the Netherlands as an au pair, and I never left! My goal was to learn Dutch, and I did. I was able to study after being in the Netherlands for three years, and I was about to graduate within the four-year term. I had been a good student after all!

In that summer of 2001, I was also in the early stages of a relationship based on trust, peace and romance. After only three months together I moved in because it felt so right. We were enjoying a lot of spontaneous romantic moments and trips to all kind of cities in Europe. On my birthday, on the 16th of July, my boyfriend gave me the most romantic and unexpected present I'd ever had. We were in Rotterdam, where we were living, dining on the terrace at Hotel New York, on a glorious summer's day. And I remember it like yesterday!

'I have something to tell you,' he said in a serious tone. So serious that I thought he had bad news to tell me. I couldn't reply, and my eyes were wide open, looking at him questioningly.

'Well, congratulations!' he said, a broad grin slowly spreading across his face.

'For what?' I asked, surprised and confused. And then he announced:

'You've been accepted! In September you'll start working at Ormit!'

'What?!?'

'Yes, I called Sandra, from the HR office, and although you were supposed to find out next week, I explained I wanted to surprise you with the good news for your birthday. She loved the idea so much that she told me.'

I was crying with joy. I was so happy. Since the previous week when I spent a full assessment day in Ormit's offices in Utrecht I had prayed to be accepted, and although *I just knew* that I would be, I didn't expect to receive the answer that way. And it was a truly fantastic way to find out! Even today, this was the most delightful and romantic surprise of my life.

That was July 2001. The brightest month of the summer and possibly the most brilliant of my life. I had been a good student, and now I had been selected because they saw my potential. Life was pure bliss.

Until a phone call from my brother turned my world and everything I knew upside down.

On the 25th of August 2001, a date that I'll never forget, I was finalising my doctoral thesis and excited about finishing it. It would be ready by the end of the month, just in time to start working at Ormit in September.

While sitting in front of my computer at the dark brown colonial wooden table in our home, working on my thesis, the phone rang. It was my brother, calling from France.

'Hi! How are you?' I asked.
'I'm not OK. Are you sitting?' He paused. He started to cry. 'It's papa. He has cancer. He's gonna die. You must come now!'

My head was spinning. I was 26 years old, my brother 23, and our younger brother wasn't even 20 yet. Our father was still young at 52. And in that moment, on what was otherwise a beautiful day of the summer of 2001, my world came crashing down. It would forever be the worst, most painful and unexpected announcement of our lives.

Death

When our grandfather passed away in 1998, he was almost 91 years old, and we knew he wouldn't make it much longer. It was the only death we had experienced until now, and it was expected. But death, as it was coming to us that day, was something else. It was about to turn my beliefs and understanding of death into complete disarray. Something was happening to me that would radically change the way I saw, understood, and thought about life.

That day, I shut down my computer on my almost finished thesis, and it would be another year before I would open it again.

That day, I wasn't sad, but I felt lost. I cried immensely and didn't know anything anymore.

That day, I wasn't scared, but I was terrified.

That day was the first of a series of long 9.5 hour drives from Rotterdam to Toulouse.

That day, while facing up to Death, was the beginning of my awakening to Life.

The next day I was in Toulouse. The imminent death of my father was confirmed. His cancer was too advanced to be cured, and he would leave us very soon, anywhere from three to six months the doctor said. Yet it would be another seven months before he departed.

One day while in Toulouse, I decided to go to the bookstore and ask what I thought would be the weirdest question that wouldn't have an answer. Still, I needed to know. I was never exposed to any literature about death, so couldn't imagine what I was about to discover.

'Hi, can I ask you a question?' I asked the lady in the bookstore.
'Yes,' she said.
'I don't even know how to ask actually... it's about my father, he has cancer and is going to die and...'
'Sure! Follow me!'

Really? Did she actually get me? I was so curious to see where she would take me.

To my surprise, she *did* get me, guiding me to a row full of books from Elisabeth Kübler-Ross, Osho, Deepak Chopra and many more. I bought several of them. And they were the first books about Death that helped me open up to Life. Maybe the most impressive lectures were those of Elisabeth Kübler-Ross, a Swiss-born American psychiatrist who pioneered the concept of providing psychological counselling to the dying. In the books I read, she was sharing her discoveries from working with terminally ill children. Her way to present Death as a full part of Life helped me accept it and also helped me wake up to life.

In her work, Elisabeth Kübler-Ross described five stages she believed were experienced by those nearing death—denial, anger, bargaining, depression, and acceptance. Observing my father, I found those steps to be accurate and clear. But further on, I started to see the similarities between Life and Death when it came to our existence and everything contained within it, and also Life and Death of all existence in a much higher perspective.

Everything around us is born and dies. Even our solar system has a beginning and will know an end. I started to ask myself *if everything has a beginning and an end, do I not have the power for allowing certain things to be birthed and to die?* I was at the time referring to my pain and suffering as I faced Death through the loss of my father. I realised my experiences would also go through different phases and eventually die. They were formed following an emotion that also popped up at one point and ended at another. The emotion is in itself a relatively brief conscious experience but my reaction to it, and its duration, is entirely up to me. And this is precisely where my power is!

My reactions are my choice and mine alone. Like an incredible motivational coach taught me when I was at Ormit: 'If it's up to be, it's up to me'!

I love to call this power 'The Power of *Creaction.*' *Creaction* is the process of choosing which *reaction* to have on an emotion, followed by an *action* that will *create* a desired outcome.

When I lost my father, I went through a huge roller coaster of emotions, sadness being the emotion that lasted the longest (up to 5 days). It is difficult to react to sadness or take action to help us get over it fast. Mourning is a process, and the grief it involves must be addressed, like all other emotions. I knew that, and I allowed myself time. Time in itself isn't a healer. It is what you do in the given time frame that will bring healing or not. If you decide to give yourself time to heal, be aware of how you choose to fill that time. If you look for the learnings and the positive side of things, then healing becomes faster and more effective. If you do not deny the mourning and its suffering and instead look at and lean into all of the darkness, your only way out will be to the Light. This unequivocally applied to me. And I know that if I'd stayed in victim mode, crying to myself, refusing to see any 'benefits' from this dark side of my experience, I'd never be where I am today.

For me, losing my father has been the catalyst for opening myself to spirituality because Death is a transition state of the soul. You see, I didn't receive any religious education. I was born in France, a secular country, in a Jewish family. Except for going to dinner during the holidays, I never gained much from the significance of it. Nevertheless, I understood one thing from being Jewish: I was different from others in my village because of a religion that I didn't choose. I wasn't allowed to join the catechism class my classmates were going to on Wednesday and share the fun they seemed to have there. For me, religion was synonymous with exclusion. However, this non-education allowed me the freedom to choose my spiritual Path.

I never believed in God as an entity outside of myself, and I refused to see God as something that would control me or decide what was good or bad. I rejected the idea of fearing consequences after death as a result of good or bad behaviour in this life. For a very long time, I saw God as the personification of a creative force bigger than ourselves. I saw 'God' as a name given by religions to an invisible power they would appropriate to themselves so they would use it to control people (especially the Catholic Church I knew from home). Even though I refused this idea of a God, I always believed in an Invisible Power in my own way.

This Invisible Power emanates from me and every other human being. A power that makes it possible for every single *being* - every existing physical particle on the planet - to effect its environment and therefore the whole world. The power behind the Butterfly effect, or the Ripple effect, you name it. I call this Invisible Power: Energy. And this energy is a movement of frequencies in space and time that is a fundamental part of our existence. Therefore I would even say that Energy *is* Life.

Confronting Death was the start of my understanding of the meaning of life. And if Death is a transition state of our soul, then what is Life about for our soul? Another transition state?

I like that idea!

'We are not human beings having a spiritual experience. We are spiritual beings having a human experience.' Most of us have heard these words from the French philosopher, Pierre Teilhard de Chardin.

What if the human experience of our Spirit, our Soul, was simply God *transitioning*? What if our lives, all those souls that chose to be in the experience of being human at this time were part of the evolution of God itself?

It's been 15 years since my father transitioned to the other side, and it has been 15 years of experiencing his presence differently. I have discovered many spiritual concepts during my spiritual journey. I've been shown many sides, many directions, many forms and heard many names (Readings, Akashic Record, Reiki, Yoga, Meditation, Prayers, Dimensions, Intergalactic Councils, etc...). But they all have one thing in common: they remind me of my connection with the Invisible Power, and I am made aware of where I am coming from and from who I am.

Doubting, feeling disconnected, unaligned, disempowered, alone, miserable and unworthy or being sad is all part of evolution's game. Never forget the goal: remember who you are.

I am *one*, and therefore I am you, you are me, and we are *all one* and not alone.

I am the energies as well as the frequencies, and therefore I have an *immense power*!

I am the incarnation of God, the Universal Creation Power, and therefore I am *free*.

I am part of God's evolution, and therefore I am *perfect*.

Author Bio:

Audrey aka The Light Coach helps you reconnect with your own light so that you can live your life in alignment, in connection with your inner voice, being guided by your heart.

Audrey has lived for a long time doing what was expected of her, truly believing she was on the right path, but she was never satisfied. She knew that she wasn't doing what really fulfilled her. So what needed to happen, happened: the breakdown and its inevitable darkness. BUT... she persisted and found her own Light! And now she's here to help you do the same, because to be faster where you belong, you simply can't do the work alone. To be the Light that you truly are and become the Lightworker you are meant to be, you need to work with someone who sees you, who feels you, who hears you, and who knows you.

Connect with Audrey:

Website: www.audreymichele.com

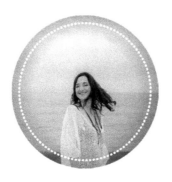

Ignite Your Inner Power
By Moni Rodriguez

'I try to live in a little bit of my own joy and not let people steal it or take it.' ~ *Hoda Kotb*

If you'd told me a year ago that I would end my second marriage, I would have thought *you* were the crazy one. Yet it happened, and very quickly. On the outside, I had the perfect relationship and enviable life, yet my soul was saying otherwise, calling me to grow and evolve, and nudging me closer to my truth.

Something inside me awakened. Something that I couldn't ignore. Something that was beckoning me to step into my authentic power, a power that, for a long time, I had diminished.

Giving our Power Away

You are crazy. You are stupid. You are ugly.

At some point in my life, I heard all these words, and I believed them. ALL of them. I let them define me for a long time, unconsciously repeating them over and over in my mind on a daily basis. I gave my power away the moment I decided that the abuse and opinions of others was true.

We are what we believe we are. And after years of listening to those voices, I decided to shift my reality and acknowledge that I am incredible just as I am. Today I feel full of love for myself and others around me. Unconditionally. The change in perception happened after a great deal of pain, fear and inner work before finally surrendering to something bigger than myself.

I had reached a point in my life whereby I'd had enough of listening to any other voices other than my own. I stopped seeking validation. I decided to walk the path of love and to claim my inner Power. The journey had begun.

We believe from a young age that we are the labels and opinions that others force on us, allowing their perceptions to define us. The reality is, we are perfect as we already are. We don't need to 'fix' or 'change' anything. We simply need to *remember* our true essence.

As Marianne Williamson once said, 'our greatest fear is not that we are inadequate. Our greatest fear is that we are powerful beyond measure.'

Not only is this universal truth, but also something that has prevented us from shining our real essence on the world. Until *now*. We *are* love. We *are* light. We are magical souls that came here to dance free; expansive, joyful and full of creativity.

But somewhere along the way, we sold our souls to the illusion. We allowed fear to take the reign. We started to feel shame, worry, and anger. We learned to suppress them, too afraid to be seen as weak, unworthy, or less than, hiding the parts of ourselves that would show others - and prove to ourselves - that we weren't good enough. Yet the mind chatter continued, and no matter what façade we wore on the outside, the voices of doubt and negativity would continue to eat away from the inside.

As a collective, we allowed external factors to hold power and control over us. Government, family, the education system - all developed by the patriarchy to keep us small and prevent us from shining our light. And as mirrors of the collective consciousness, we became controlling too. We wanted to control our relationships, our children, our emotions, everything. We created resistance. We locked the door and lost the key to our freedom.

Now we have been called to unlock the door. To open our heart and allow our soul to flourish and dance free.

Now, let me warn you: following and fully opening your heart is not always easy. It is in complete contrast to how you were conditioned, requiring you to shed the false perception of power. Real power comes from surrender, and being authentically and unapologetically you. Embracing your light and loving your shadow, forgiving yourself for all the pain and abuse you have suffered directly or indirectly. And the adventure never ends. The journey doesn't have any clear destination. The destination is the journey itself. In any given moment, you are precisely where you need to be.

The journey of healing is infinite; it doesn't end. Ultimately, we came here to learn how to love - ourselves and each other - in unity. To love our shadow *and* our light. To integrate and bring into harmony our masculine and feminine aspects of self. And it requires a commitment to faith, to listening to your intuition, and most importantly the voice of your heart.

What is your Truth?

The decision to end my second marriage was not easy. To be honest, I hadn't seen it coming. My soul was taking a quantum leap, awakening something in me like never before. Something fierce. Honest. Magnificent. The pure truth inside was waiting and ready to be expressed. The pain and sorrow that came with it were beyond my comprehension. I couldn't believe that I was on the edge of something new once more and in the process of total transformation that would shatter my illusions and everything that I'd believed to be true. The more I loved myself, and the more I was getting to know myself, the more clarity I gained about unconditional love, relationships and my spiritual path.

I found myself in a place of total confusion with my reality until I let myself hear the real voice of my soul. I openly spoke with my (now) ex, and without finding a way back or seeking resolution, I moved forward with the changes I knew I had to make. As I always do, I followed my intuition and my heart: the decision to end my marriage was what followed.

Leaving everything you once knew as 'safe' is not easy. It's pretty damn hard even if you are full of courage and as adaptable to change as I am. Despite always holding joy in my heart, it didn't make it any less painful.

In my experience, when we get comfortable with people and our environment, we create a false sense of safety and identity. To me, we can't feel truly safe or experience love until we go back home to our heart and we find true love in unity inside ourselves.

Following your truth is the only thing that is real. We can pretend everything is just 'fine', but if the soul wants to evolve, it will always start crying until you don't have any other choice than to face it. You can make it harder for yourself trying to ignore it, continuing to live what feels like a double-life. Or you can confront your fears and find the courage to step up and free yourself from any limitations that you have created.

In my experience, each of us comes here to learn our lessons. Each expression is unique as are the lessons for each of us.

What connects us all is that we came here to walk the path of love in one way or another. For me, my true power comes with unconditional love and compassion for myself and others, and from actualising my creative gifts. When we connect with our true soul essence, we feel whole, complete, at peace and free.

Walking the path of love requires a tremendous amount of courage and faith. The journey will bring you pain as you look into your shadows, recognising the parts that feel lost and empty, feeling overwhelmed by the desire to change.

When you are ready, you know. You won't be able to deny it any longer.

You will recognise that you can't stop crying, feeling sad, flat and experiencing waves of grief without apparent reason. The feeling that something is wrong will haunt you; it will feel inescapable. You will get a sense that there is something better on the other side of all of your fear, yet you won't be able to see what it is. You will be ready to seek, but at the same time, you will feel scared. *What if I fail? What If I deceive myself? Why can't I be 'normal'? Am I selfish?* All these questions will hammer away at your mind. You will feel like your entire world is falling apart with a nagging sense of urgency being the only constant.

The time will come, and you will know.

Feel the Pain, Learn the Lessons

Walking the path of love within yourself requires you to transmute energy and heal parts of you that feel 'broken'. The truth is that you were never broken; you simply forgot the way home. The way to your heart is a path that you walk when you decide to face the fears inside you. *All* of them. Allow yourself to feel all the emotions that come up in your journey and in silence, ask them: *what do you want me to know?* Eventually, if you are quiet enough, you will receive an answer. You must allow yourself to feel the pain completely. Surrender to it, and let it engulf you. You will hear the truth inside you about what needs to be transmuted.

During my recent journey I experienced a lot of anger. One day the anger was so intense that I couldn't think clearly. Tired of feeling this way I intuitively asked the anger: *'What are you trying to tell me?'* To my surprise, I immediately received a response. *'I am tired of feeling oppressed.'* I continued asking *'oppressed by what?'* The answer came back again: *'To express myself freely.'* I delved further: *'What can you do to express yourself more freely?'* And then the magical moment came: *'By Expressing yourself and your essence even more.'*

It was then that I understood the lesson that my anger was bringing; I no longer felt the need to suppress it or feel bad for how I was feeling. In that moment I felt an immense fire in my belly. I knew I had transmuted my feelings and I had a burning passion that wanted to be expressed in many ways: dancing, writing, singing and doing even more loving things for myself.

I invite you to do the same when negative emotions creep into your life. Ask them for the lesson that they are here to teach. Look for the gift in their presence. And remember: the choice is *always* yours. Do you choose to unconditionally love yourself and others? Or do you let fear rule your world?

Be brave dear one. We only live once. Make it worth it. Let your soul dance free. Enjoy the journey.

Author Bio:

#1 International Best-Selling Author, Speaker and Coach, Moni helps women around the world transform stress and overwhelm into greater peace, passion and joy.

Currently based in London and originally from the beautiful city of Barcelona, Moni, otherwise known as Monica, believes that when women shine their light and claim their inner power, they can change the world.

With more than 15 years of experience in corporate Moni has observed that a more compassionate and heart-centred leadership is required to bring back balance, equality and consciousness.

She is passionate about banishing burnout from the corporate culture, and is committed to supporting women lead projects. Moni is helping and inspiring women around the world to transform their life and become leaders for change in both their personal and professional lives.

With her writing, signature talks and support, Moni contributes to raising awareness of increasing the presence of feminine values in the world.

Connect with Moni:

Website: www.monirodriguez.com
Instagram/twitter/FB/pinterest: @monirodriguezsp

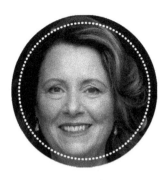

Giving my Power Away
By Denise Davis

'The more fears we walk through, the more power we reclaim' ~ Robin Sharma

Have you ever acted so entirely different to what you expected? I did. You see, I always imagined that if my husband left me, I'd either cling onto him, crying and begging him to stay, or unleash fistfuls of fury if he admitted infidelity. Well, neither of those scenarios happened. Instead, I felt numb.

Looking back I'd always feared men. I was petrified of my violent father as a child. I often stood rooted to the spot, overtly aware of his volatility, knowing he could turn at any moment, wetting myself in fear and silent anticipation. I was a very quiet and shy unobtrusive kid, always blending into the background, unlike my siblings who were bolder, louder, and would challenge him. He left when I was eleven, yet the hold he still had over me was palpable. He was physically strong, someone to fear, always in control; his mere presence shook me to the core of my being.

At age nine I learned that I was a sexual object. I'd often stay at a neighbour's house and play with their son. One night while sleeping he touched my budding breasts. I stiffened. I knew it didn't feel right, that it was wrong, yet I didn't know what to do. So I accepted it. Said nothing. Simply made excuses not to sleep over again while meeting up and acting as normal during the day.

At thirteen a male teacher took a shine to me. I looked older for my age. Being the eldest of four kids with a full-time working and single mum meant that I took on a lot of the responsibility of my siblings; I had to grow up fast. My teacher, despite being married with a baby on the way, started asking me out to places and bought me gifts and cards. Initially, I was flattered as all the girls at school fancied him (including me). I felt noticed. Wanted. Loved. My low self-esteem given a much-needed boost. There were many times that he kept me behind for 'detention' so that he could spend time with me. Again I was very passive and didn't know how to extricate myself.

After a while, the lies and subterfuge became too much for me, and I finally got the courage to end the 'relationship.' However by this time he told me his wife knew and was going to cite me in their divorce case. Yet more fear. More silence.

I became like honey to a bee with men, a taste that was, for me, bittersweet. Men who were old enough to know better. Men who propositioned me. Friends. Neighbours husbands. Men whose children I'd just spent the evening babysitting. Every encounter, every interaction, I laughed off politely, too afraid to stand my ground.

My step-dad was brought into our home when I was fourteen. He decided that he wanted to be my first sexual encounter, despite the fact I already had a boyfriend (or that he was in a relationship with my mother). Somehow I managed to get out of that one although to this day I'm unable to recall how.

The same boyfriend and I got engaged when I was sixteen. He was three years older and very jealous and possessive. It's hard for me to look back and see how desperate for love I was that I could allow so much emotional and physical abuse. I recall one time when he pinned me up against the wall and gripped my throat so hard I could hardly breathe. And I thought that was love!!

Meeting my husband soon after was like a breath of fresh air. He was nothing like any of the men I'd met previously. He was kind, thoughtful and attracted to the feistiness that I'd developed to protect myself. I made it clear that I wouldn't have sex with him until I was ready. This was one boundary I had set and adhered to throughout my teens. I loved that he made me laugh and we got on well on many levels. After six months we were engaged and by our first year together had booked the church for our wedding.

Happily Ever After

We had to bring the wedding forward as I fell pregnant despite being careful. My future mother-in-law was ashamed and embarrassed about what to tell others. I too felt embarrassed but decided that my baby was a gift from God – our love child. By the time we had our second child mortgage prices had risen so much that we decided to start a new life in Doha, Qatar.

In Doha I opened my own small school while expecting my third child. It was an eye-opener; an entirely new way of life. Here I was surrounded by material wealth, people (apparently) free of worry and concern who could enjoy the finer things in life. They worked hard, but they played harder.

Shortly after my daughter was born my mother died unexpectedly and so we flew back to England for the funeral. I was inconsolable. In shock. She seemed so young at fourty-nine and had been a picture of health when I'd seen her only months before. I sought solace in my old church, seeking comfort and guidance. Yet all faith was lost when the vicar advised that my mum was now in hell because of her lack of commitment to the church, despite her devotion to God all her life.

Feeling lost and confused my younger sister and I decided to visit a medium. My mum came through. I felt immense relief and reassurance that she was okay; the medium even gave us evidence by reciting some of our conversation from that afternoon. My spiritual doorway had begun to open.

When I told my husband, he was agitated and angry, ordering me not to do anything like this again. Spirituality wasn't in his realm of thinking; he was scared. Of course I slipped into old patterns, allowing myself to be controlled by a man and did exactly as he'd asked. With four kids, studying for my degree, working and running the household, I was exhausted. And while I desperately wanted to explore my spirituality I believed that keeping my husband happy by following his wishes made for an easier and quieter life.

Keeping the Peace & Giving up on Dreams

Throughout my entire marriage I played small, dimming my light to appease my husband. I gave up my power, allowed him and everyone else to decide and dictate what was right for me.

At eighteen I couldn't play tennis because my wrists were supposedly too small.

I wasn't 'allowed' to scuba dive or paraglide because it was allegedly unsafe.

I suspect he didn't want to be burdened with young kids on his own while I dared to enjoy myself, although he never actually justified anything to me, simply gave a very firm no.

Slowly I was curling up and dying inside! Not fully growing and exploring my world in a physical and metaphysical sense. On the outside I was bright and bubbly, befitting the role of a corporate wife and primary school teacher. Yet on the inside my self-worth was shot to pieces and my marriage crumbling with it.

D-Day

I still loved my husband. But it wasn't reciprocated. I spent days crying and feeling desperate, confused, lost, ashamed, humiliated and wounded. I still wanted his warmth, his comfort, in spite of everything, yet was faced with coldness and rejection. One minute he wanted me, the next he didn't. We'd act like a couple then he'd make it clear that it was purely platonic.

It took nine long months of purgatory knowing that my husband could leave at any moment before the day came that he finally said goodbye and this time it was me calling the shots.

I was so exhausted emotionally and physically that I eventually asked him to leave. He wanted more time but I refused. I could no longer cope with it all. He left that weekend. I stood at the front door, handing him his clothes. I felt numb.

That summer a family member told me they had seen him with another woman. I didn't believe it. I couldn't. I assumed that being the mother of his children he'd afford me the decency to tell me himself. Of course he didn't. And it was true. I said to him that everyone deserves to be happy, that he shouldn't feel guilty blah blah blah. Yet when I got home after our meeting, the floodgates opened and I started to grieve.

The hurt. The anger. The pain. The abandonment. The betrayal.

I grieved the holidays we'd never have, the years that went into raising our children.

I grieved every single memory that would be forgotten, good and bad.

I grieved the parts of me that I'd given up, neglected and abandoned, to keep *him* happy.

Life After Divorce

My life changed radically. I was no longer teaching and my kids had flown the nest. I delved into my passions and interests. I explored floristry, healing and coaching. I decided to have FUN. I partied, went dancing and drinking, busied my mind and filled up my diary to distract me from the pain that I was numbing myself from. I put on a mask yet felt crushed and devastated on the inside.

Yet I now found myself free to explore my spirituality again. And after attending a workshop and being told that I was clairsentient and an empath, my interest was reignited! I started to attend a spiritualist church where at the end of the service a woman told me that I had healed her. The penny dropped. My eyes opened. I suddenly looked back at my life and the people I'd met and the experiences I'd had. Why people would tell me their life story without any encouragement, why I always felt others pain, sadness and joy and so tried to prevent incurring anymore for them. And why I never told anyone about the way men treated me because of the pain I was trying to avoid causing others. I subsequently discovered that my grandmothers on both my father's and mother's side had been healers and seers too. For the first time in my life, I felt free. I felt that I knew who I was, why I was here and suddenly my whole purpose of being fell into place.

I've since delved into my psychic development, training in many different healing and therapy techniques. I've shifted from a place of self-lack and oppression to self-love and care. I completed a tandem freefall skydive with my youngest son when I was 50 followed by finally doing the PADI scuba diving certificate I had wanted to do when living in Doha. I've traveled the world for fun and adventure as well as to train and professionally develop. I also followed my heart and moved to Dorset, somewhere I had wanted to live since returning from Qatar. I leaped into the unknown by moving to where I didn't know a single soul, yet had a deeper knowing that my life would be happier somehow. I stepped out of my comfort zone, attended events and groups and now have a wonderful life filled with friendship, fun, learning and being of service as a Coach.

I'm free in many ways now and finally accept and love the person I am, putting myself first (most of the time) and realising that at sixty, if I didn't do things for myself now, then when would I. Life is a gift. We are meant to live it in the present moment, for ourselves. May you follow your inner guidance to create a life of freedom and choice, loving and honouring yourself along the way for your frailties and strengths.

Reader Notes:

Where in life have you allowed others to dictate how you live your life?

Do you have firm boundaries in place or are you easily persuaded by others to change your mind?

Have you ever celebrated your achievements and how far you have come?

Do you realise that your inner guidance is the only thing that will keep you on the right track - when things 'feel' right then you are good to go. Contrariwise if things feel 'off' don't do them!

Author Bio:

Denise Davis works with children and adults so they become more of who they truly are. She will teach you how to harmonise your heart and live your life with more control, confidence and charisma, so that you feel relaxed, rebalanced and rejuvenated. This enables you to reach more of your potential as you have left behind some of your limiting beliefs, have greater work life balance, with more self-awareness and emotional intelligence.

Denise brings you back to the essence of you - having reignited your connection with your inner guidance which helps you create a life of choice, joy and authenticity thus living your life more fully.

She does this through one to one sessions, workshops and talks. Denise is qualified in many coaching and healing modalities and the latest addition to her toolkit is a bio resonance machine which helps your body repair itself and return to equilibrium.

Denise lives in Dorset by the sea and the new forest. She loves being in nature. Denise loves spending time with friends and family having lots of fun and laughter. She has four children and five grandchildren so far, whom she adores... a puppy and more are a couple of her plans for the future.

Connect with Denise:

Facebook page: Harmonise Your Heart
Twitter: @dee_lightful1
Skype: dee-lightful1
Instagram: @denisedavis123

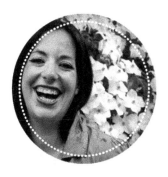

Turning your Sensitivity into your Superpower
By Kara Grant

'Never be ashamed to let your tears shine a light in this world.' ~ Anthon St. Maarten

I became a people-pleaser when I met a man I loved.

Up until then, my twenties were full of toxic, broken relationships that ravished my sense of worth and value. I didn't fit whatever preconception I had of a woman who had been abused. Outwardly I was confident, I was functioning, I had a good life, and I appeared happy. But I didn't like myself, at all. In fact, even the relationship I went back to *after* I was date-raped by him still wasn't as toxic as the one I was in with myself.

I hit that dark place. I was training to be a Yoga teacher, and during meditation, I had a flashback to childhood abuse. My breakdown/breakthrough was tough. But I had finally sorted my shit out. I started therapy and discovered the techniques and way of living that would become my work.

Yes! I had done the work. I was 'healed'. Now I could get on with living. And I did.

But, here is the thing. My inner fear freaks were having a field day in this burgeoning new relationship. I was a mess of anxiety and paranoia. I pushed it all down. Having learned about the law of attraction, I was scared that if I admitted to any of these negative emotions, then that would become my reality.

I second-guessed everything. And put meaning upon meaning upon meaning. I remember many times my partner would make an innocuous joke and I would find myself in the bathroom crying over what I'd made everything mean.

My perfectionist came out to play. Now, we all have our very own particular brand of perfectionism. Mine will be vastly different to yours. Your inner perfectionist is the one who tells you 'no one will love you if you show you are broken or damaged'. So she is likely to stage manage a lot of the masks you wear.

You might be working ridiculous hours, forfeiting your lunch breaks and weekends to check emails and giving 110% when you are running on empty, yet your perfectionist is telling you it's still not enough. Maybe she's telling you not to cry in front of your friends or show that you're struggling and instead pretend that everything's okay. Or perhaps she's telling you to hide your past, to push it into the shadows because no-one will love you if they knew the truth.

My perfectionist was harsh, yet she was nothing compared to my people pleaser. She paved the way for my people pleaser to go wild.

I imagine they spoke to each other a little like this:

Perfectionist: 'OK, so she has found a good relationship, she needs to keep it *all* together and keep him'.
People pleaser: 'Allow me - I reckon she needs to work damn hard to suppress what she wants and needs because what she needs is dangerous and is going to leave her all on her own'.

So that's precisely what I did, and for a while, it worked. However, something I've learned is that no matter how much you hold it all together and people-please your way through life, the truth will always out.

Stepping into Truth

Sex has always been painful for me. It ranged from messy to hysterical to using self-harm as a way to channel some of the hate and disgust I felt for myself.

Until a few years ago, I either avoided sex entirely or numbed myself with alcohol to get through it. All I wanted was to be normal.

Sex with my new partner was different. It felt like love. I felt safe. I loved being so close to him. It was fun. I felt like this was what I had been looking for, this was how it was supposed to be.

But my people pleaser was there in full force. '*Don't let him know you aren't normal. He is going to think you are weird when he finds out you've never had an orgasm. And when he finds out about the abuse? That's it; you're out of there.*'

It took a while for me to tell him and if I had one wish around this for any woman who has struggled with sex or abuse, it would be for her to speak her truth from the start. Because me living a lie led to a lot of pain.

How you do one thing is how you do everything. And the parts of your true self that you hide show up in every area of your life.

As a sensitive woman if you aren't speaking your truth your Higher Self will let you know; whether you listen is another story. And how long it takes to pay attention depends on the level of discomfort and the lingering sense of unease you're willing to live with.

No matter what you've been through and how many coping mechanisms you develop, nothing is as painful (or exhausting) as suppressing who you really are. And nothing is more empowering than reclaiming your inner power.

I remember the moment that I realised that I had to let go of everything I knew to live in truth and integrity of who I really was.

By this point, I had a gorgeous man, a beautiful little boy (Arthur) and a business I was proud of. I was happy. But my Higher Self kept telling me: 'You aren't living your truth.'

And I wasn't. This complicated way of living that I had created to please my partner was exhausting.

Besides, no one had told me to live this way. No one had forced me to wear a mask and live a lie; it was all my creation. At some point, I'd decided that that was how life was meant to be, yet along the way, I forgot that I was responsible for my life, for my happiness.

Slowly my partner and I started to argue more. Scott knew I wasn't honest with him. He desperately wanted me to open up yet felt stonewalled when I didn't. I felt his frustration, and it angered me. *Who the hell did he think he was feeling annoyed when I was the one battling my inner fear freaks every day?* Tensions were high and to add to that we were living with his parents. I felt like I had no space; I was a pressure-cooker of emotion ready to explode. I decided to visit Scotland. I found a place to stay for a week on my own with Arthur.

Scott asked: 'Do you want me to come up with you?'

I panicked. This was going to be space for me. I needed to be on my own. I didn't want him there, but I couldn't say no. And I felt guilty, like I was abandoning him, rejecting him, pushing him away.

'Do you want to?' There I was again, unable to speak my truth. I was so angry with myself. *That* was the moment. I saw his hurt expression and knew what I needed to say. 'No. I need space.'

The resulting conversation was so hard, and I felt terrible for letting it get to that point. But in another way, I'm glad it did. For me, it had to get to *that* point, that moment for me to breathe through Scott's hurt, something that would typically trigger my need to please, to understand I couldn't live that way.

The time away was what I needed. My people pleaser had told me I wouldn't be accepted if I asked for what I needed but I felt nothing but the deepest support from Scott during the whole period.

I realised that I could still be loved when I asked for what I wanted. In fact, I *was* loved when I asked for what I needed.

You will be loved, and you will be safe when you ask for what you need, I promise.

Ditching the People Pleaser

In that week away I spent my son's nap times meditating. The evenings were spent writing in my journal and a long letter to my partner

The moment I spoke my truth was the moment I let go of the power my people pleaser had over me, but there were still more and more layers to unpeel.

I had to let go of expecting my partner to make me happy and the unhealthy co-dependency I had created.

When your people pleaser sees someone you love hurt she goes into a tailspin. But when the hurt is caused by letting go of people pleasing you have no option but to ride the discomfort out. It starts with a decision and a whole lot of trust that it will all work out.

When I share about the people pleaser with my clients and in the Sisterhood, it resonates with a *lot* of women. There seems to be two ways women arrive at people-pleasing: through learned behaviour at a very young age or, like me, as a coping mechanism for self-protection. There are times when I wish I were still back in that place of not owning my behaviour. In so many ways that feels easier, right?

But it isn't. It is a vacuum keeping you stuck.

What I have recognised is that sensitive woman all identify with the people pleaser. These women are women who want to bring real change into the world.

They have a massive capacity for love: giving and receiving. If you are reading this chapter, I know that's you too. You have so much within you. And you want to have the most intimate and abundant life.

I hear you. Because that's me too. And now, I can live my desired life because I ditched my attachment to my people pleaser. And once you ditch your people pleaser? You're ready to unleash your sensitivity as your superpower.

Owning your Sensitivity as your Superpower

My priorities changed when I owned my Sensitivity as my Superpower. I am a work in progress; I will be for life. And there is still so much I'm learning. What I do know right now is that overwhelm is my Achilles heel.

Overwhelm is one of the biggest stressors when you are a sensitive superstar. It is *so* easy to fall into overwhelm. It is addictive and all-consuming. I had to become a warrior of my well-being, which means I don't do *anything* that will contribute to my feelings of overwhelm. Writing this makes me recognise how huge this is for me. No longer feeling tied to anyone's agenda or be at the mercy of what you are hearing and seeing and no longer engulfed in a tidal wave of fear is the most freeing expression for a sensitive superstar. Two things happened to get me there:

1) I own being sensitive. I don't defend myself if I feel emotional. I don't feel the need to explain. I understand myself so much more. When I first got therapy following my abuse memory, I learned about loving and appreciating myself. But that was the first level. It goes way *deeper*. It needs to be done on a cellular level when

you *know* yourself. You understand the way your emotions impact you, what triggers you and your monthly cycle. My God. Learning about my period and hormones has to be one of the most empowering decisions I've made in my life to date. Knowing where I am in my cycle and how my hormones might be influencing my emotions, stress-levels and outlook is permission to be *all* of me. It also gives me the responsibility to take ownership and do what I need to de-stress and balance my emotions. Or the permission to sack it all off and go to bed if that's what I need!

2) I became the warrior of my well-being. My emotional well-being is my priority. I am a driven person, driven by impact and connection. However, when I get caught up in this drive, I can easily neglect my emotional well-being and slip into overwhelm.

And what brings these two together is my practice.

Your Practice as your Lifeline

My practice is my lifeline. When I need it, it's there. When I wake up in the morning, it is my way to connect with my Higher Self. When I need guidance, inspiration and answers, it supports me. Whether that's meditation, yoga, running, walking or dancing for you – as a sensitive superstar, it's your life-blood. When you make it a priority, ensuring that your needs are met, life becomes expansive, filled with love, compassion and peace.

Owning your sensitivity as your superpower will not stop you being emotional, it will enable you to process, surrender and empower yourself. It will mean your gorgeous lion heart can roar with love and compassion, firstly towards yourself and then to the world around you. Owning your sensitivity as your superpower will not stop you feeling bad. Instead, it will support you in moving back into peace and joy. But owning your sensitivity as your superpower *will* create the intimacy and abundance and freedom you crave. Go on superstar; it's your time.

Reader Notes:

1) Take some deep breaths and journal around these questions:

   Do I feel I am speaking my truth?
   Do I feel I own my sensitivity as a superpower?
   Where in my life am I people pleasing?

Then write down 1-3 micro aligned actions that will support you with moving closer to feeling more empowered and free in your life.

2) To help you when you are in overwhelm:

Suggested Mantra: You can say this anytime you go into overwhelm. Take some really deep breaths, breathing into the belly as you inhale and releasing as you exhale:

'I trust I am more than enough'

Author Bio:

Kara is a writer, coach + speaker. She believes that sensitive women are here to change the world. As founder of the Sensitive Sisterhood she has created a space for sensitive women to come together in community and be supported to bring their gifts into the world while living their desired life.

An award winning entrepreneur, Kara loves sharing her story and hearing other women sharing theirs too. She is delighted to be part of the Uncaged project and be surrounded by amazing women who are using their voices for change.

Kara lives in Manchester with her boys. She loves spending time under the stars at festivals and having adventures in the sun.

Connect with Kara:

FB: www.facebook.com/sensitivesuperstars
Instagram: www.instagram.com/karavgrant

Ready to join the #WomenRise movement?

Share your story on Instagram and tag @riseofthebadass & @michelle_catanach

Join our #WomenRise Facebook group.